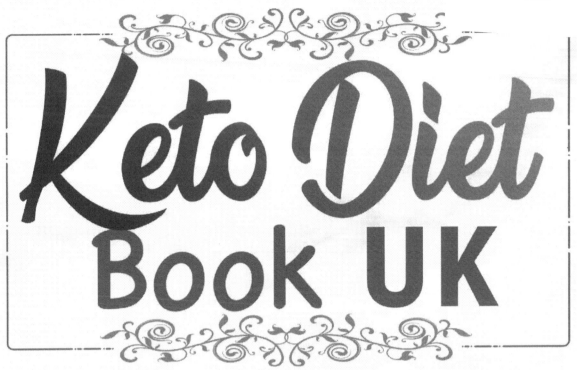

Keto Diet Book UK

The Complete Keto Diet Cookbook with Quick and Healthy Recipes

Dr. Daniel Smith

INTRODUCTION...**7**

What is the Keto Diet? 7

How does Keto Diet work? 7

Different types of Keto iDiets 8

What is ketosis? 9

Ketogenic diets can help you lose weight 9

Ketogenic diets for diabetes and prediabetes 10

Other health benefits of keto 10

Foods to avoid 11

Foods to eat 11

Healthy keto snacks 11

Keto tips and tricks 12

Tips for eating out on a ketogenic diet 12

Side effects and how to minimize them..12

Supplements for a ketogenic diet 13

The bottom line 13

THE 35 DAY MEAL PLAN... **14**

First Week Meal Plan 15

Second Week Meal Plan 16

Third Week Meal Plan..17

Fourth Week Meal Plan..18

Fifth Week Meal Plan...19

Breakfast Recipes.. **20**

Keto-Styled Scrambled Eggs..20

Avocado Coconut Milk Shake...20

Lemon Fried Avocados 21

Keto Butter Coffee 22

Mexican egg roll..22

Baked Eggs...23

Veggie breakfast bakes 24

Scrambled eggs with basil and butter 24

Keto Boosted Coffee 25

Keto deviled eggs 25

Keto mushroom omelet 26

Tomato baked eggs 27

Spicy keto deviled eggs 28

Keto oven-baked Brie cheese 28

Keto Coffee Recipe 29

Easy Seed & Nut Granola 29

Keto fried halloumi cheese with mushrooms 30

Egg and Ham Rolls 31

Keto cheese omelet 31

Coconut oil Coffee 32

Keto smoked salmon plate 33

Almond Butter Choco Shake 33

Lunch Recipes **34**

Goat cheese salad with balsamico butter 34

Hearty Cauliflower, Leek & Bacon Soup 35

Keto Blueberry Smoothie 35

Prosciutto-wrapped salmon skewers 36

Keto tuna plate 37

Strawberry Avocado Smoothie 37

Keto smoked salmon and avocado plate 38

Green Keto Smoothie 38

Broccoli Bacon Salad 39

Chicken Nuggets 40

Peanut Butter Smoothie 40

Keto salmon-filled avocados 41

Keto salmon and spinach plate 42

Keto Flu Smoothie 42

Chicken Bacon Burgers 43

Keto Smoothie Recipe 43

Basil Chicken Saute 44

Crispy Chicken Drumsticks 44

Keto Avocado Brownies 45

Keto mackerel and egg plate 46

Keto fried salmon with green beans 46

Guacamole Burgers 47

Easy Broccoli Beef Stir-Fry 48

Keto fried salmon with broccoli 48

Keto fried salmon with asparagus 49

Keto baked salmon with lemon and butter 50

Pan-Fried Pork Tenderloin 51

Rosemary Baked Salmon 51

Keto ground beef and green beans 52

Keto ground beef and broccoli 53

Keto turkey plate 53

Cucumber Ginger Shrimp 54

Dinners Recipes **55**

Keto Cream Cheese Pancake 55

Keto oven-baked chicken in garlic butter 55

Keto fried chicken with cabbage 56

Turkey Arugula Salad 57

Keto fried chicken with broccoli and butter 57

Cumin Crusted Lamb Chops 58

Nut Free Keto Brownie 59

Keto chicken pesto 59

Cheese, Mortadella and Salami 60

Keto chicken and green beans plate 61

Keto chicken and Feta cheese plate 61

Keto chicken and cabbage plate 62

Mushroom brunch 63

Herb omelette with fried tomatoes 63

Egg with Bacon & Asparagus Soldiers 64

Soft-boiled eggs with pancetta avocado 65

Gordon's eggs Benedict 65

Lamb & lettuce pan-fry 66

Chilli avocado 67

Italian keto plate 67

Keto fried salmon with broccoli and cheese 68

Keto Ground Beef Enchiladas 68

Grilled Buttermilk Chicken 69

Pistachio Salmon 70

Sauteed Radishes with Green Beans 70

Zucchini Noodles 71

Bonus Recipes **72**

Grilled Peppered Steaks 72

Grilled Lemon-Garlic Salmon 72

Buffalo Pulled Chicken 73

Cheesy Roasted Broccoli 74

Quick Garlic-Lime Chicken 74

Keto Fat Bombs 75

Oven-Roasted Salmon 76

Ham Pickle Pinwheels 76

Coconut Crack Bars 77

Lemon-Butter Tilapia with Almonds 78

Keto Pancakes 78

Cream Cheese Muffins 79

Keto Palmini Spaghetti Bolognese 80

Mashed Cauliflower with Chives 81

Garlic Parmesan Zucchini 81

Mashed Cauliflower with Chives 82

Keto ground beef and green beans 83

Low-carb baked eggs 83

Butter Hardboiled Eggs 84

Creamy Avocado Cacao Chia Shake 84

Crispy-Fried Wings 85

Perfect Family Roast 86

Peanut Butter Chia Pudding 86

Salted Toffee Walnut Cups 87

Keto Milk Chocolate 88

No-Bake Keto Cookies 89

Caprese Salad 89

Cream Cheese Crepes 90

Cauliflower Bake 90

Zucchini Tomato Soup 91

Easy Keto Ice Cream 92

Scrambled Eggs with Bacon 92

Crispy Chicken Wings 93

Kale Chips 94

Keto Pizza Chips 94

Chia Seeds Smoothie 95

Feta Cheese Omelet 95

Sausage and Eggs 96

Easy Bacon and Eggs 96

Surprise Recipes **97**

Chicken Curry 97

Easy Baked Chicken Breast 98

Garlic Chicken 98

Rosemary Chicken and Bacon 99

Grilled Turkey Burgers 99

Spicy Chicken Wings 100

Juicy Beef Tenderloin 100

Easy Pork Steaks 101

Pure Indulgence Peanut Butter Biscuits 102

Craftily Creamy Chocolate Mousse 102

Chewy Coconut Chunks 103

Keto chicken enchilada bowl 103

Healthy Lunchtime Ham & Cheese Wrap 104

Cheesy Chicken Chunks 104

Creamy Avocado Cilantro 105

Spain Cheesy-Meat Tapas 106

Tasty Salted Turnip Fries 106

Overnight Oats 107

CONCLUSION **107**

INTRODUCTION

Hello! Thanks for purchasing this book, "The Complete Keto Diet Book UK"
The Ketogenic diet is not like others kinds of diet through which you will lose weight quickly, but then gain it back. The diet is a scientifically proven method to lose weight. The diet allows dieters to lose weight without having to count calories. One of the main reasons why the diet works well is that this diet doesn't restrict your calorie intake. You can enjoy your favorite foods with the Ketogenic diet instead of avoiding them.

What is the Keto Diet?

The ketogenic diet is based on using fat, rather than carbohydrates, as the primary source of energy. The diet is designed to result in ketosis, a state in which your body produces a molecule called ketones from fat molecules that you eat. Ketones, instead of glucose, become the primary energy molecule in your body. The ketogenic diet can aid in weight loss because, as your body becomes adapted to burning fat as fuel, it draws upon body fat reserves rather than burning carbohydrates and storing excess energy as fat. The ketogenic diet was first developed as a treatment for drug resistant epilepsy about one hundred years ago and is still used as one of the most effective treatments for a range of seizure disorders. Over time, doctors noticed that other physiological effects resulted from this diet. Potential benefits from following the ketogenic diet include weight loss, better appetite control, increased and more consistent energy levels, better insulin sensitivity, treatment of insulin-related disor- ders like diabetes, and fewer damaging effects from high or highly variable blood glucose levels. The standard ketogenic diet entails extreme carbohydrate restriction, with carbohydrates accounting for 3-5% of total calories, protein supplying 7-10%, and fat supplying 85-90%. This is very hard to follow and is mostly used in clinical settings. The modified ketogenic diet offers many of the same benefits with greater flexibility. Carbohydrates supply 5-13% of calories, protein supplies 15-30%, and fat supplies 60 to 80%, with saturated fat supplying no more than 20% of total calories.

How does Keto Diet work?

A ketogenic diet is one in which carbohydrate intake is severely restricted. However, not all low-carbohydrate diets are ketogenic. There are three approaches to low-carb eating, and only one of them is considered a proper keto diet. On a ketogenic diet, your body goes into a state of ketosis, where it burns fat as fuel. This process produces ketones, which gives these diets their "keto" name. On most ketogenic diets, you consume 70 to 75 percent of your calories from fat. Of the remainder, you consume about 5 to 10 percent of your calories from carbohydrates and the rest from protein. However, there is some variation in the structure of the diet. Some sources say to consume no more than 20 grams of carbohydrates per day, while others cite up to 50 grams, and many recommend no more than five percent of calories from carbs.

Meals are most often built around fat sources such as fatty fish, meat, nuts, cheese, and oils. Some versions of the keto diet advise that you eat only certain types of fat. For example, many authors recommend steering clear oils that are high in polyunsaturated omega-6 fats (soy, corn, cottonseed, safflower) because they are considered to be less healthy. Some diet foods recommend fats high in medium-chain triglycerides (MCT), such as coconut oil and MCT oil, as these fats are quickly turned into ketones by the body.

In general, people on ketogenic diets tend to consume many foods high in monounsaturated and saturated fats such as olive oil, butter (from grass-fed cows is recommended), avocado, and cheeses. The high oleic types of safflower and sunflower oils (but not the common forms of these oils) are often recommended. They are high in monounsaturated fats and low in polyunsaturated fats.

While there is no need to time meals, purchase specific products, or eat individual required snacks or beverages, the diet does not provide much flexibility in terms of food choice because carbohydrates are so severely restricted.

Different types of Keto Diets

There are several versions of the ketogenic diet, including:

- **The standard ketogenic diet (SKD)** is a very low carb, moderate protein, and high-fat diet. It typically contains 70% fat, 20% protein, and only 10% carbs (9Trusted Source).

- **The cyclical ketogenic diet (CKD):** This diet involves periods of higher-carb refeeds, such as five ketogenic days followed by two high carb days.

- **The targeted ketogenic diet (TKD):** This diet allows you to add carbs around workouts.

- **High protein ketogenic diet:** This is similar to a standard ketogenic diet but includes more protein. The ratio is often 60% fat, 35% protein, and 5% carbs.

However, only the standard and high protein ketogenic diets have been studied extensively. Cyclical or targeted ketogenic diets are more advanced methods and are primarily used by bodybuilders or athletes.

What is ketosis?

Ketosis is a metabolic state in which your body uses fat for fuel instead of carbs.

It occurs when you significantly reduce your consumption of carbohydrates, limiting your body's supply of glucose (sugar), which is the main source of energy for the cells.

Following a ketogenic diet is the most effective way to enter ketosis. Generally, this involves limiting carb consumption to around 20 to 50 grams per day and filling up on fats, such as meat, fish, eggs, nuts, and healthy oils.

It's also important to moderate your protein consumption. This is because protein can be converted into glucose if consumed in high amounts, which may slow your transition into ketosis.

Practicing intermittent fasting could also help you enter ketosis faster. There are many different forms of intermittent fasting, but the most common method involves limiting food intake to around 8 hours per day and fasting for the remaining 16 hours.

Blood, urine, and breath tests are available, which can help determine whether you've entered ketosis by measuring the amount of ketones produced by your body.

Certain symptoms may also indicate that you've entered ketosis, including increased thirst, dry mouth, frequent urination, and decreased hunger or appetite.

Ketogenic diets can help you lose weight

A ketogenic diet is an effective way to lose weight and lower risk factors for disease.

In fact, research shows that the ketogenic diet may be as effective for weight loss as a low-fat diet.

What's more, the diet is so filling that you can lose weight without counting calories or tracking your food intake.

One review of 13 studies found that following a very low carb, ketogenic diet was slightly more effective for long-term weight loss than a low-fat diet. People who followed the keto diet lost an average of 2 pounds (0.9 kg) more than the group that followed a low-fat diet.

What's more, it also led to reductions in diastolic blood pressure and triglyceride levels.

Another study in 34 older adults found that those who followed a ketogenic diet for 8 weeks lost nearly five times as much total body fat as those who followed a low-fat diet.

The increased ketones, lower blood sugar levels, and improved insulin sensitivity may also play a key role.

Ketogenic diets for diabetes and prediabetes

Diabetes is characterized by changes in metabolism, high blood sugar, and impaired insulin function.

The ketogenic diet can help you lose excess fat, which is closely linked to type 2 diabetes, prediabetes, and metabolic syndrome.

One older study found that the ketogenic diet improved insulin sensitivity by a whopping 75%.

A small study in women with type 2 diabetes also found that following a ketogenic diet for 90 days significantly reduced levels of hemoglobin A1C, which is a measure of long-term blood sugar management.

Another study in 349 people with type 2 diabetes found that those who followed a ketogenic diet lost an average of 26.2 pounds (11.9 kg) over a 2-year period. This is an important benefit when considering the link between weight and type 2 diabetes.

What's more, they also experienced improved blood sugar management, and the use of certain blood sugar medications decreased among participants throughout the course of the study.

Other health benefits of keto

The ketogenic diet actually originated as a tool for treating neurological diseases such as epilepsy.

Studies have now shown that the diet can have benefits for a wide variety of different health conditions:

Heart disease: The ketogenic diet can help improve risk factors like body fat, HDL (good) cholesterol levels, blood pressure, and blood sugar.

Cancer: The diet is currently being explored as an additional treatment for cancer, because it may help slow tumor growth.

Alzheimer's disease: The keto diet may help reduce symptoms of Alzheimer's disease and slow its progression.

Epilepsy: Research has shown that the ketogenic diet can cause significant reductions in seizures in epileptic children.

Parkinson's disease: Although more research is needed, one study found that the diet helped improve symptoms of Parkinson's disease.

Polycystic ovary syndrome: The ketogenic diet can help reduce insulin levels, which may play a key role in polycystic ovary syndrome.

Brain injuries: Some research suggests that the diet could improve outcomes of traumatic brain injuries.

However, keep in mind that research into many of these areas is far from conclusive.

Foods to avoid

Any food that's high in carbs should be limited.

Here's a list of foods that need to be reduced or eliminated on a ketogenic diet:

- sugary foods: soda, fruit juice, smoothies, cake, ice cream, candy, etc.
- grains or starches: wheat-based products, rice, pasta, cereal, etc.
- fruit: all fruit, except small portions of berries like strawberries
- beans or legumes: peas, kidney beans, lentils, chickpeas, etc.
- root vegetables and tubers: potatoes, sweet potatoes, carrots, parsnips, etc.
- low fat or diet products: low fat mayonnaise, salad dressings, and condiments
- some condiments or sauces: barbecue sauce, honey mustard, teriyaki sauce, ketchup, etc.
- unhealthy fats: processed vegetable oils, mayonnaise, etc.
- alcohol: beer, wine, liquor, mixed drinks
- sugar-free diet foods: sugar-free candies, syrups, puddings, sweeteners, desserts, etc.

Foods to eat

You should base the majority of your meals around these foods:

- meat: red meat, steak, ham, sausage, bacon, chicken, and turkey
- fatty fish: salmon, trout, tuna, and mackerel
- eggs: pastured or omega-3 whole eggs
- butter and cream: grass-fed butter and heavy cream
- cheese: unprocessed cheeses like cheddar, goat, cream, blue, or mozzarella
- nuts and seeds: almonds, walnuts, flaxseeds, pumpkin seeds, chia seeds, etc.
- healthy oils: extra virgin olive oil, coconut oil, and avocado oil
- avocados: whole avocados or freshly made guacamole
- low carb veggies: green veggies, tomatoes, onions, peppers, etc.
- condiments: salt, pepper, herbs, and spices

Healthy keto snacks

In case you get hungry between meals, here are some healthy, keto-approved snacks:

- fatty meat or fish
- cheese
- a handful of nuts or seeds
- keto sushi bites
- olives
- one or two hard-boiled or deviled eggs

- keto-friendly snack bars
- 90% dark chocolate
- full-fat Greek yogurt mixed with nut butter and cocoa powder
- bell peppers and guacamole
- strawberries and plain cottage cheese
- celery with salsa and guacamole
- beef jerky
- smaller portions of leftover meals
- fat bombs

Keto tips and tricks

Although getting started on the ketogenic diet can be challenging, there are several tips and tricks that you can use to make it easier.

- Start by familiarizing yourself with food labels and checking the grams of fat, carbs, and fiber to determine how your favorite foods can fit into your diet.
- Planning out your meals in advance may also be beneficial and can help you save extra time throughout the week.
- Many websites, food blogs, apps, and cookbooks also offer keto-friendly recipes and meal ideas that you can use to build your own custom menu.
- Alternatively, some meal delivery services even offer keto-friendly options for a quick and convenient way to enjoy keto meals at home.
- Look into healthy frozen keto meals when you're short on time
- When going to social gatherings or visiting family and friends, you may also want to consider bringing your own food, which can make it much easier to curb cravings and stick to your meal plan.

Tips for eating out on a ketogenic diet

Many restaurant meals can be made keto-friendly.

Most restaurants offer some kind of meat or fish-based dish. Order this and replace any high carb food with extra vegetables. Egg-based meals are also a great option, such as an omelet or eggs and bacon. Another favorite is bun-less burgers. You could also swap the fries for vegetables instead. Add extra avocado, cheese, bacon, or eggs.

At Mexican restaurants, you can enjoy any type of meat with extra cheese, guacamole, salsa, and sour cream.

For dessert, ask for a mixed cheese board or berries with cream.

Side effects and how to minimize them

Although the ketogenic diet is usually safe for most healthy people, there may be some initial side effects while your body adapts. There's some anecdotal evidence of these effects often referred to as the keto flu (38Trusted Source). Based on reports from some on the eating plan, it's usually over within a few days.

Reported keto flu symptoms include diarrhea, constipation, and vomiting (39Trusted Source). Other less common symptoms include:

- poor energy and mental function
- increased hunger
- sleep issues
- nausea
- digestive discomfort
- decreased exercise performance

To minimize this, you can try a regular low carb diet for the first few weeks. This may teach your body to burn more fat before you completely eliminate carbs. A ketogenic diet can also change the water and mineral balance of your body, so adding extra salt to your meals or taking mineral supplements may help. Talk to your doctor about your nutritional needs. At least in the beginning, it's important to eat until you're full and avoid restricting calories too much. Usually, a ketogenic diet causes weight loss without intentional calorie restriction.

Supplements for a ketogenic diet

Although no supplements are required, some can be useful.

- MCT oil: Added to drinks or yogurt, MCT oil provides energy and helps increase ketone levels. Shop for MCT oil online.
- Minerals: Added salt and other minerals can be important when starting out due to shifts in water and mineral balance.
- Caffeine: Caffeine can have benefits for energy, fat loss, and performance (45).
- Exogenous ketones: This supplement may help raise the body's ketone levels.
- Creatine: Creatine provides numerous benefits for health and performance. This can help if you are combining a ketogenic diet with exercise.
- Whey: Use half a scoop of whey protein in shakes or yogurt to increase your daily protein intake. Shop for tasty whey products on online.

The bottom line

A ketogenic diet can be great for people who:

- are overweight
- have diabetes
- are looking to improve their metabolic health

It may be less suitable for elite athletes or those wishing to add large amounts of muscle or weight.

It may also not be sustainable for some people's lifestyles and preferences. Speak with your doctor about your eating plan and goals to decide if a keto eating plan right for you.

THE 35 DAY MEAL PLAN

Now, the moment you've been waiting for — the meal plan! In this chapter, you'll find a 35-day meal plan for the standard ketogenic diet, divided into four weeks. Every day you'll follow the plan to eat breakfast, lunch, and dinner, as well as a snack or dessert with a calorie range between 1,800 and 2,000.

One thing I want to mention before you get started is net carbs.

Many people who follow the ketogenic diet prefer to track net carbs rather than total carbs. To calculate net orbs, you simply take the total carb count of the meal and subtract the grams of fiber since fiber cannot be digested. Personally. I prefer to track total carbs like what I have mentioned in my first book, but I have included the grams of fiber and net carbs in these recipes, so you can choose which way to go.

personally, I prefers more buffer when it comes to the carb count, because I want to reduce the number of obstacles keeping me from ketosis. Many of my readers as well as friends have raised this point and you can be sure quite a few nights or afternoons were spent in heated debate! Okay, it wasn't that serious but suffice it to say that quite a bit of discussion went into this topic Therefore, I thought it might be better if I gave you a say in this net carb-total orb debate. You get to choose whichever you prefer. In my personal opinion, when you are in the initial stages of trying to enter ketosis, keeping your total carb count in mind is probably one of the better practices you can adopt. A 20 to 50gram range of carbs would usually work to push the body into a ketogenic state.

After you have gotten keto adapted and the body gets used to burning fat for fuel, you on then start to bring net carbs into the equation.

Keep in mind the calorie range for these meal plans — if you read my first book and calculated your own daily caloric needs, you may need to make some adjustments. If you're trying the ketogenic diet for the first time, however, it may be easiest to just follow the plan as is until you get the hang of it.

The first week of this 35-day meal plan is designed to be incredibly simple in terms of meal prep so wan can focus on learning which foods to eat and which to avoid on the ketogenic diet — that's why you'll find more smoothies and soups here than in the following weeks. If you finish the first week and feel like you still need some time making the adjustment to keto, feel free to repeat it before moving on to week two. The meal plans also take into account left-overs and the yields of various recipes, so that you have minimal wage from your efforts in the kitchen. So, without further ado, let's take a look at the meal plans

35-Days Keto Diet Weight Loss Challenge

First Week Meal Plan

Day	Breakfast	Lunch	Dinner
Sunday	Keto Butter Coffee (Page No. 22)	Broccoli Bacon Salad (Page No. 39)	Keto fried chicken with cabbage (Page No. 56)
Monday	Keto Boosted Coffee (Page No. 25)	Keto Blueberry Smoothie (Page No. 35)	Soft-boiled eggs with pancetta avocado (Page No. 65)
Tuesday	Coconut oil Coffee (Page No. 32)	Strawberry Avocado Smoothie (Page No. 37)	Keto fried chicken with broccoli and butter (Page No. 57)
Wednesday	Keto Butter Coffee (Page No. 22)	Broccoli Bacon Salad (Page No. 39)	Keto fried chicken with cabbage (Page No. 56)
Thursday	Keto Boosted Coffee (Page No. 25)	Keto Blueberry Smoothie (Page No. 35)	Soft-boiled eggs with pancetta avocado (Page No. 65)
Friday	Coconut oil Coffee (Page No. 32)	Strawberry Avocado Smoothie (Page No. 37)	Keto fried chicken with broccoli and butter (Page No. 57)
Saturday	Coconut oil Coffee (Page No. 32)	Strawberry Avocado Smoothie (Page No. 37)	Keto fried chicken with broccoli and butter (Page No. 57)

35-Days Keto Diet Weight Loss Challenge

Second Week Meal Plan

Day	Breakfast	Lunch	Dinner
Sunday	Keto Coffee Recipe (Page No. 29)	Keto Flu Smoothie (Page No. 42)	Keto chicken and cabbage plate (Page No. 62)
Monday	Tomato baked eggs (Page No. 27)	Keto Smoothie Recipe (Page No. 43)	Herb omelette with fried tomatoes (Page No. 63)
Tuesday	Keto Coffee Recipe (Page No. 29)	Keto Flu Smoothie (Page No. 42)	Keto chicken and cabbage plate (Page No. 62)
Wednesday	Tomato baked eggs (Page No. 27)	Keto Smoothie Recipe (Page No. 43)	Herb omelette with fried tomatoes (Page No. 63)
Thursday	Keto Coffee Recipe (Page No. 29)	Keto Flu Smoothie (Page No. 42)	Keto chicken and cabbage plate (Page No. 62)
Friday	Keto Coffee Recipe (Page No. 29)	Keto Flu Smoothie (Page No. 42)	Keto chicken and cabbage plate (Page No. 62)
Saturday	Tomato baked eggs (Page No. 27)	Keto Smoothie Recipe (Page No. 43)	Herb omelette with fried tomatoes (Page No. 63)

35-Days Keto Diet Weight Loss Challenge

Third Week Meal Plan

Day	Breakfast	Lunch	Dinner
Sunday	Keto Butter Coffee (Page No. 22)	Keto Smoothie Recipe (Page No. 43)	Herb omelette with fried tomatoes (Page No. 63)
Monday	Coconut oil Coffee (Page No. 32)	Keto Blueberry Smoothie (Page No. 35)	Zucchini Noodles (Page No. 71)
Tuesday	Keto Butter Coffee (Page No. 22)	Keto Smoothie Recipe (Page No. 43)	Herb omelette with fried tomatoes (Page No. 63)
Wednesday	Coconut oil Coffee (Page No. 32)	Keto Blueberry Smoothie (Page No. 35)	Zucchini Noodles (Page No. 71)
Thursday	Keto Butter Coffee (Page No. 22)	Keto Smoothie Recipe (Page No. 43)	Herb omelette with fried tomatoes (Page No. 63)
Friday	Coconut oil Coffee (Page No. 32)	Keto Blueberry Smoothie (Page No. 35)	Zucchini Noodles (Page No. 71)
Saturday	Keto Butter Coffee (Page No. 22)	Keto Smoothie Recipe (Page No. 43)	Herb omelette with fried tomatoes (Page No. 63)

35-Days Keto Diet Weight Loss Challenge

Fourth Week Meal Plan

Day	Breakfast	Lunch	Dinner
Sunday	Keto Boosted Coffee (Page No. 25)	Keto Smoothie Recipe (Page No. 43)	Chilli avocado (Page No. 67)
Monday	Keto Butter Coffee (Page No. 22)	Keto Flu Smoothie (Page No. 42)	Zucchini Noodles (Page No. 71)
Tuesday	Keto Boosted Coffee (Page No. 25)	Keto Smoothie Recipe (Page No. 43)	Chilli avocado (Page No. 67)
Wednesday	Keto Butter Coffee (Page No. 22)	Keto Flu Smoothie (Page No. 42)	Zucchini Noodles (Page No. 71)
Thursday	Keto Boosted Coffee (Page No. 25)	Keto Smoothie Recipe (Page No. 43)	Chilli avocado (Page No. 67)
Friday	Keto Butter Coffee (Page No. 22)	Keto Flu Smoothie (Page No. 42)	Zucchini Noodles (Page No. 71)
Saturday	Keto Boosted Coffee (Page No. 25)	Keto Smoothie Recipe (Page No. 43)	Chilli avocado (Page No. 67)

35-Days Keto Diet Weight Loss Challenge

Fifth Week Meal Plan

Day	Breakfast	Lunch	Dinner
Sunday	Keto Boosted Coffee (Page No. 25)	Keto Flu Smoothie (Page No. 42)	Chilli avocado (Page No. 67)
Monday	Keto Boosted Coffee (Page No. 25)	Keto Blueberry Smoothie (Page No. 35)	Keto chicken and cabbage plate (Page No. 62)
Tuesday	Keto Boosted Coffee (Page No. 25)	Keto Flu Smoothie (Page No. 42)	Chilli avocado (Page No. 67)
Wednesday	Keto Boosted Coffee (Page No. 25)	Keto Blueberry Smoothie (Page No. 35)	Keto chicken and cabbage plate (Page No. 62)
Thursday	Keto Boosted Coffee (Page No. 25)	Keto Flu Smoothie (Page No. 42)	Chilli avocado (Page No. 67)
Friday	Keto Boosted Coffee (Page No. 25)	Keto Blueberry Smoothie (Page No. 35)	Keto chicken and cabbage plate (Page No. 62)
Saturday	Keto Boosted Coffee (Page No. 25)	Keto Flu Smoothie (Page No. 42)	Chilli avocado (Page No. 67)

Breakfast Recipes

Keto-Styled Scrambled Eggs

Prep. Time: 05 min

Cook Time: 05 min

Servings: 1 People

Ingredients

- 1 tbsp of unsalted butter
- 3 Large Eggs
- Coarse salt & freshly ground pepper

Instruction

1. Beat together the eggs using a fork.
2. In a medium nonstick pan, melt the butter over low heat.
3. Add the egg mixture.
4. Use a heatproof flexible spatula to pull the eggs gently to the center of the skillet. *Let the liquid parts run out under the perimeter*.
5. Cook, keep moving eggs around using the spatula for 2-3 minutes, just until the eggs are set.
6. Add salt and pepper to season. Serve hot.

Nutrition Per Servings: Kcal: 318, Protein: 17g, Fat: 26g, Net Carb: 1.8g

Avocado Coconut Milk Shake

Prep. Time: 05 min

Cook Time: 00 min

Servings: 1 People

Ingredients

- ½ avocado
- ½ cups Unsweetened Coconut Milk
- 5 drops stevia
- 5 Ice Cubes

Instruction

1. Add all the ingredients to the blender. Blend until smooth.

Nutrition Per Servings: Kcal: 437, Protein: 5g, Fat: 43g, Net Carb: 10g

Bulletproof Coffee

Prep. Time: 05 min

Cook Time: 00 min

Servings: 1 People

Ingredients

- 1 tbsp MCT Oil
- 2 tbsp Butter
- 12 oz Coffee

Instruction

1. Brew a cup of coffee using any brewing method you'd like.
2. Add butter, MCT oil, and coffee to a blender. Blend on high for 30 seconds. Enjoy.

Nutrition Per Servings: Kcal: 320, Protein: 0g, Fat: 36g, Net Carb: 0g

Lemon Fried Avocados

Prep. Time: 02 min

Cook Time: 05 min

Servings: 2 People

Ingredients

- 1 ripe avocado (not too soft), cut into slices
- 1 Tablespoon (15 ml) coconut oil
- 1 Tablespoon (15 ml) lemon juice
- Salt to taste (or lemon salt)

Instruction

1. Add coconut oil to a frying pan. Place the avocado slices into the oil gently.
2. Fry the avocado slices (turning gently) so that all sides are slightly browned.
3. Sprinkle the lemon juice and salt over the slices and serve warm.

Nutrition Per Servings: Kcal: 200, Protein: 02g, Fat: 20g, Net Carb: 2g

Keto Butter Coffee

Prep. Time: 05 min

Cook Time: 00 min

Servings: 1 People

Ingredients

- 1 cup of water
- 2 tbsp coffee
- 1 tbsp grass-fed butter
- 1 tbsp coconut oil

Instruction

Make a cup of coffee in your favourite way. We like to use Turkish Coffee Pot. We simply simmer ground coffee in water for about 5 minutes and then strain it into our cup. You can also use a Moka Pot, a French press, or a coffee machine!

1. Pour your brewed coffee into your blender (like a Nutribullet) and butter and coconut oil. Blend for about 10 seconds. You'll see it instantly become light and creamy!
2. Pour the butter coffee into a mug and enjoy! Add in any other ingredients you'd like in this step like cinnamon or whipped cream!

Nutrition Per Servings: Kcal: 230, Protein: 0g, Fat: 25g, Net Carb: 0g

Mexican egg roll

Prep. Time: 5 min

Cook Time: 10 min

Servings: 2 People

Ingredients

- 1 large egg
- a little rapeseed oil for frying
- 2 tbsp tomato salsa
- about 1 tbsp fresh coriander

Instruction

1. Beat the egg with 1 tbsp water. Heat the oil in a medium non-stick pan. Add the egg and swirl round the base of the pan, as though you are making a pancake, and cook until set. There is no need to turn it.
2. Carefully tip the pancake onto a board, spread with the salsa, sprinkle with the coriander, then roll it up. It can be eaten warm or cold – you can keep it for 2 days in the fridge.

Nutrition Per Servings: Kcal: 132, Protein:10g, Fat: 9g, Net Carb: 1g

Baked Eggs

Prep. Time: 10 min

Cook Time: 35 min

Servings: 2 People

Ingredients

- 4 Eggs
- 4 Slices Bacon
- Salt and Pepper to taste 1 Oz Cheddar
- 1 Small Onion (80g)

Instruction

1. Fry four slices of bacon
2. Cut a small onion in half and fry
3. In a ramekin or equivalent oven-proof bowl, place onion and bacon
4. Crack two eggs into each container, making sure to not break yolk
5. Add salt and pepper
6. Add cheddar cheese
7. Bake at 350 degrees for 20 minutes or until eggs have set

Nutrition Per Servings: Kcal: 338, Protein: 21g, Fat: 24g, Net Carb: 5g

Veggie breakfast bakes

Prep. Time: 10 min

Cook Time: 40 min

Servings: 4 People

Ingredients

- 4 large field mushrooms
- 8 tomatoes , halved
- 1 garlic clove , thinly sliced
- 2 tsp olive oil
- 200g bag spinach
- 4 eggs

Instruction

1. Heat oven to 200C/180C fan/gas 6. Put the mushrooms and tomatoes into 4 ovenproof dishes. Divide garlic between the dishes, drizzle over the oil and some seasoning, then bake for 10 mins.
2. Meanwhile, put the spinach into a large colander, then pour over a kettle of boiling water to wilt it. Squeeze out any excess water, then add the spinach to the dishes. Make a little gap between the vegetables and crack an egg into each dish. Return to the oven and cook for a further 8-10 mins or until the egg is cooked to your liking.

Nutrition Per Servings: Kcal: 127, Protein: 09g, Fat: 08g, Net Carb: 05g

Scrambled eggs with basil and butter

Prep. Time: 05 min

Cook Time: 10 min

Servings: 2 People

Ingredients

- 4 tbsp butter
- 4 eggs
- 4 tbsp heavy whipping cream
- salt and ground black pepper
- 4 oz. shredded cheese

- 4 tbsp fresh basil

Instruction

1. Melt butter in a pan on low heat.
2. Add cracked eggs, cream, shredded cheese, and seasoning to a small bowl. Give it a light whisk and add to the pan.
3. Stir with a spatula from the edge towards the center until the eggs are scrambled. If you prefer it soft and creamy, stir on lower heat until desired consistency.
4. Top with fresh basil.

Nutrition Per Servings: Kcal: 625, Protein: 40g, Fat: 60g, Net Carb: 4g

Keto Boosted Coffee

Prep. Time: 02 min

Cook Time: 00 min

Servings: 16 People

Ingredients

- 2 cup freshly brewed hot coffee
- Two tablespoons grass-fed butter
- One scoop Perfect Keto MCT Powder
- One teaspoon Ceylon cinnamon

Instruction

1. Combine all of the ingredients in a blender.

Nutrition Per Servings: Kcal: 625, Protein: 40g, Fat: 60g, Net Carb: 4g

Keto deviled eggs

Prep. Time: 05 min

Cook Time: 10 min

Servings: 2 People

Ingredients

- 2 eggs

- ½ tsp tabasco
- 2 tbsp mayonnaise
- ½ pinch herbal salt
- 4 cooked and peeled shrimp
- fresh dill

Instruction

1. Start by boiling the eggs by placing them in a pot and covering them with water. Place the pot over medium heat and bring to a light boil.
2. Boil for 8-10 minutes to make sure the eggs are hardboiled.
3. Remove the eggs from the pot and place in an ice bath for a few minutes before peeling.
4. Split the eggs in half and scoop out the yolks.
5. Place the egg whites on a plate.
6. Mash the yolks with a fork and add tabasco, herbal salt and homemade mayonnaise.
7. Add the mixture, using two spoons, to the egg whites and top with a shrimp on each, or a piece of smoked salmon.
8. Decorate with dill.

Nutrition Per Servings: Kcal: 170, Protein: 08g, Fat: 16g, Net Carb: 1g

Keto mushroom omelet

Prep. Time: 05 min

Cook Time: 15 min

Servings: 2 People

Ingredients

- 6 eggs
- 2 oz. butter, for frying
- 2 oz. shredded cheese
- ½ yellow onion, chopped
- 8 large mushrooms, sliced
  salt and pepper

Instruction

1. Crack the eggs into a mixing bowl with a pinch of salt and pepper. Whisk the eggs with a fork until smooth and frothy.

2. Melt the butter in a frying pan, over medium heat. Add the mushrooms and onion to the pan, stirring until tender, and then pour in the egg mixture, surrounding the veggies.
3. When the omelet begins to cook and get firm, but still has a little raw egg on top, sprinkle cheese over the egg.
4. Using a spatula, carefully ease around the edges of the omelet, and then fold it over in half. When it starts to turn golden brown underneath, remove the pan from the heat and slide the omelet on to a plate.

Nutrition Per Servings: Kcal: 230, Protein: 16g, Fat: 21g, Net Carb: 2g

Tomato baked eggs

Prep. Time: 10 min

Cook Time: 50 min

Servings: 4 People

Ingredients

- 900g ripe vine tomatoes
- 3 garlic cloves
- 3 tbsp olive oil
- 4 large free range eggs
- 2 tbsp chopped parsley and/or chives

Instruction

1. Preheat the oven to fan 180C/ conventional 200C/gas 6. Cut the tomatoes into quarters or thick wedges, depending on their size, then spread them over a fairly shallow 1.5 litre ovenproof dish. Peel the garlic, slice thinly and sprinkle over the tomatoes. Drizzle with the olive oil, season well with salt and pepper and stir everything together until the tomatoes are glistening.
2. Slide the dish into the oven and bake for 40 minutes until the tomatoes have softened and are tinged with brown.
3. Make four gaps among the tomatoes, break an egg into each gap and cover the dish with a sheet of foil. Return it to the oven for 5-10 minutes until the eggs are set to your liking. Scatter over the herbs and serve piping hot with thick slices of toast or warm ciabatta and a green salad on the side.

Nutrition Per Servings: Kcal: 204, Protein: 09g, Fat: 16g, Net Carb: 4g

Spicy keto deviled eggs

Prep. Time: 10 min

Cook Time: 10 min

Servings: 6 People

Ingredients

- 6 eggs
- 1 tbsp red curry paste
- ½ cup mayonnaise
- ¼ tsp salt
- ½ tbsp poppy seeds

Instruction

1. Place the eggs in cold water in a pan, just enough water to cover the eggs. Bring to a boil without a lid.
2. Let the eggs simmer for about eight minutes. Cool quickly in ice-cold water.
3. Remove the egg shells. Cut off both ends and split the egg in half. Scoop out the egg yolk and place in a small bowl.
4. Place the egg whites on a plate and let sit in the refrigerator.
5. Mix curry paste, mayonnaise and egg yolks into a smooth batter. Salt to taste.
6. Bring out the egg whites from the refrigerator and apply the batter.
7. Sprinkle the seeds on top and serve.

Nutrition Per Servings: Kcal: 200, Protein: 06g, Fat: 19g, Net Carb: 1g

Keto oven-baked Brie cheese

Prep. Time: 05 min

Cook Time: 10 min

Servings: 4 People

Ingredients

- 9 oz. Brie cheese or Camembert cheese
- 1 garlic clove, minced
- 1 tbsp fresh rosemary, coarsely chopped
- 2 oz. pecans or walnuts, coarsely chopped
- 1 tbsp olive oil

salt and pepper

Instruction

1. Preheat the oven to 400°F (200°C).
2. Place the cheese on a sheet pan lined with parchment paper or in a small non-stick baking dish.
3. In a small bowl, mix the garlic, herb and nuts together with the olive oil. Add salt and pepper to taste.
4. Place the nut mixture on the cheese and bake for 10 minutes or until cheese is warm and soft and nuts are toasted. Serve warm or lukewarm.

Nutrition Per Servings: Kcal: 342, Protein: 15g, Fat: 31g, Net Carb: 1g

Keto Coffee Recipe

Prep. Time: 07 min

Cook Time: 10 min

Servings: 4 People

Ingredients

12 oz freshly brewed coffee

1-2 tbsp Butter

1/4 tsp liquid stevia

Instruction

1. Add all ingredients to a blender jar and blend for 10 seconds.

Carefully remove the lid and pour into a coffee mug. See notes for other blending options.

Nutrition Per Servings: Kcal: 200, Protein: 1g, Fat: 22g, Net Carb: 0g

Easy Seed & Nut Granola

Prep. Time: 05 min

Cook Time: 00 min

Servings: 5 People

Ingredients

- Small handful of nuts (10 almonds, 3 Brazil nuts, 5 cashews)
- 2 Tablespoons (17 g) pumpkin seeds
- 1 Tablespoon (12 g) cacao nibs
- 1 Tablespoon (5 g) coconut flakes
- 1/4 cup (60 ml) unsweetened coconut or almond milk

Instruction

1. Mix together all the dry ingredients. If you're making a large batch, then store leftovers in an airtight container. Serve with coconut or almond milk.

Nutrition Per Servings: Kcal: 400, Protein: 09g, Fat: 30g, Net Carb: 09g

Keto fried halloumi cheese with mushrooms

Prep. Time: 05 min

Cook Time: 10 min

Servings: 2 People

Ingredients

- 10 oz. mushrooms
- 10 oz. halloumi cheese
- 3 oz. butter
- 10 green olives
- salt and pepper

Instruction

1. Rinse and trim the mushrooms, and cut or slice.
2. Heat up a hearty dollp of butter in a frying pan where you can fit both halloumi cheese and mushrooms.
3. Fry the mushrooms on medium heat for 3-5 minutes until they are golden brown. Season with salt and pepper.
4. If necessary, add more butter and fry the halloumi for a couple of minutes on each side. Stir the mushrooms every now and then. Lower the heat towards the end. Serve with olives.

Nutrition Per Servings: Kcal: 830, Protein: 36g, Fat: 74g, Net Carb: 7g

Egg and Ham Rolls

Prep. Time: 10 min

Cook Time: 15 min

Servings: 4 People

Ingredients

- 4 slices of ham
- 1 cucumber, sliced thin
- 4 eggs, whisked well
- 2 Tablespoons (30 ml) avocado oil, to cook with

Instruction

1. Add 1 teaspoon of avocado oil to a frying pan on low to medium heat and spread it around with a paper towel.
2. Add 1/4 cup of whisked eggs to the pan and roll it around to spread it thin.
3. Place a lid on top of the frying pan and let it cook until the base of the egg wrap is cooked (approx. 2-3 minutes). Carefully place on a plate and let cool.
4. Repeat in batches with the rest of the egg mixture to make egg wraps.
5. Create rolls with the egg wraps, slices of ham, and cucumber slices.

Nutrition Per Servings: Kcal: 158, Protein: 12g, Fat: 13g, Net Carb: 1g

Keto cheese omelet

Prep. Time: 05 min

Cook Time: 10 min

Servings: 2 People

Ingredients

- 3 oz. butter
- 6 eggs
- 7 oz. shredded cheddar cheese
- salt and pepper to taste

Instruction

1. Whisk the eggs until smooth and slightly frothy. Blend in half of the shredded cheddar. Salt and pepper to taste.

2. Melt the butter in a hot frying pan. Pour in the egg mixture and let it set for a few minutes.

3. Lower the heat and continue to cook until the egg mixture is almost cooked through. Add the remaining shredded cheese. Fold and serve immediately.

Nutrition Per Servings: Kcal: 897, Protein: 40g, Fat: 80g, Net Carb: 4g

Coconut oil Coffee

Prep. Time: 05 min

Cook Time: 01 min

Servings: 1 People

Ingredients

- 1 cup coffee
- 1 1/2 tsp coconut oil
- 1/2 cup warm coconut milk optional
- 1/8 tsp cinnamon optional
- 1/8 tsp cayenne pepper optional
- Whole cloves for garnish
- Coconut cream for garnish
- Star anise for garnish

Instruction

1. Make a cup of coffee as you normally would and pour it into a blender.

2. Add the coconut oil to the blender and blend for 1-2 minutes until the mixture lightens in colour and becomes frothy.

3. Add any extras you'd like, including warm coconut milk, cinnamon, and or cayenne pepper, and give it a quick blend for 10-20 seconds.

4. Pour into a mug, top with coconut cream, and grind fresh cloves over the cream, if desired.

5. Garnish with star anise, and enjoy warm.

Nutrition Per Servings: Kcal: 61, Protein: 0g, Fat: 6g, Net Carb: 0.1g

Keto smoked salmon plate

Prep. Time: 05 min

Cook Time: 00 min

Servings: 2 People

Ingredients

- 12 oz. smoked salmon
- 1 cup mayonnaise
- 2 cups baby spinach
- 1 tbsp olive oil
- ½ lime (optional)
- salt and pepper

Instruction

1. Put salmon, spinach, a wedge of lime, and a hearty dollop of mayonnaise on a plate.
2. Drizzle olive oil over the spinach and season with salt and pepper.

Nutrition Per Servings: Kcal: 1016, Protein: 33g, Fat: 97g, Net Carb: 1g

Almond Butter Choco Shake

Prep. Time: 05 min

Cook Time: 00 min

Servings: 1 People

Ingredients

- 1 cup (240 ml) coconut milk or almond milk
- 2 Tablespoons (10 g) unsweetened cacao powder (or 1 scoop CoBionic Indulgence for added collagen)
- 1 Tablespoon (16 g) almond butter
- 1 teaspoon (5 ml) vanilla extract
- 1/4 cup (35 g) ice (optional)
- Erythritol or stevia to taste (optional)

Instruction

1. Place all the ingredients into a blender and blend well.

Nutrition Per Servings: Kcal: 190, Protein: 04g, Fat: 15g, Net Carb: 7g

Lunch Recipes

Goat cheese salad with balsamico butter

Prep. Time: 05 min

Cook Time: 10 min

Servings: 2 People

Ingredients

- 10 oz. goat cheese
- ¼ cup pumpkin seeds
- 2 oz. butter
- 1 tbsp balsamic vinegar
- 3 oz. baby spinach

Instruction

1. Preheat the oven to 400°F (200°C).
2. Put slices of goat cheese in a greased baking dish and bake in the oven for 10 minutes.
3. While the goat cheese is in the oven, toast pumpkin seeds in a dry frying pan over fairly high temperature until they get some color and start to pop.
4. Lower the heat, add butter and let simmer until it turns a golden-brown color and a pleasant nutty scent. Add balsamic vinegar and let boil for a few more minutes. Turn off the heat.
5. Spread out baby spinach on a plate. Place the cheese on top and add the balsamico butter.

Nutrition Per Servings: Kcal: 824, Protein: 37g, Fat: 73g, Net Carb: 3g

Hearty Cauliflower, Leek & Bacon Soup

Prep. Time: 10 min

Cook Time: 60 min

Servings: 4 People

Ingredients

- 1/2 head of cauliflower, chopped
- 6 cups (1.4 l) chicken broth or bone broth
- 1 leek, chopped
- 5 slices of bacon, cooked
- Salt and pepper to taste

Instruction

1. Place the chopped cauliflower and leek into a pot with the chicken broth.
2. Cover the pot and simmer for 1 hour or until tender.
3. Use an immersion blender to puree the vegetables to create a smooth soup. (If you don't have an immersion blender, you can take the vegetables out, let cool briefly, puree in a normal blender, and then put back into the pot.)
4. Crumble the cooked bacon into small pieces and drop into the soup.
5. Add salt and pepper to taste.

Nutrition Per Servings: Kcal: 110, Protein: 10g, Fat: 04g, Net Carb: 06g

Keto Blueberry Smoothie

Prep. Time: 05 min

Cook Time: 00 min

Servings: 1 People

Ingredients

- 1 cup Coconut Milk or almond milk
- 1/4 cup Blueberries
- 1 tsp Vanilla Extract
- 1 tsp MCT Oil or coconut oil

- 30 g Protein Powder optional

Instruction

1. Put all the ingredients into a blender, and blend until smooth.

Nutrition Per Servings: Kcal: 215, Protein: 23g, Fat: 10g, Net Carb: 5g

Prosciutto-wrapped salmon skewers

Prep. Time: 10 min

Cook Time: 15 min

Servings: 4 People

Ingredients

- ¼ cup fresh basil, finely chopped
- 1 lb salmon, boneless fillets, frozen in pieces
- 1 pinch ground black pepper
- 3½ oz. prosciutto, in slices
- 1 tbsp olive oil
- 8 wooden skewers

Instruction

1. Soak the skewers.
2. Chop the basil finely with a sharp knife.
3. Cut the almost thawed lax-filet pieces length-wise and mount on the skewers.
4. Roll the skewers in the chopped basil and pepper.
5. Slice the prosciutto into thin strips and wrap around the salmon.
6. Cover in olive oil and fry in a pan, oven or on the grill.
7. Serve with the mayonnaise or a hearty salad and a rich aioli.

Nutrition Per Servings: Kcal: 680, Protein: 28g, Fat: 62g, Net Carb: 01g

Keto tuna plate

Prep. Time: 05 min

Cook Time: 10 min

Servings: 2 People

Ingredients

- 4 eggs
- 2 oz. baby spinach
- 10 oz. tuna in olive oil
- 1 avocado
- ½ cup mayonnaise
  salt and pepper

Instruction

1. Begin by cooking the eggs. Lower them carefully into boiling water and boil for 4-8 minutes depending on whether you like them soft or hard boiled.
2. Cool the eggs in ice-cold water for 1-2 minutes when they're done; this will make it easier to remove the shell.
3. Place eggs, spinach, tuna and avocado on a plate. Serve with a hearty dollop of mayonnaise and perhaps a wedge of lemon. Season with salt and pepper.

Nutrition Per Servings: Kcal: 931, Protein: 52g, Fat: 76g, Net Carb: 03g

Strawberry Avocado Smoothie

Prep. Time: 05 min

Cook Time: 00 min

Servings: 5 People

Ingredients

- 1 lb Frozen strawberries
- 1 1/2 cups Almond Breeze Original Almond Milk (regular or vanilla)
- One large Avocado
- 1/4 cup Besti Powdered Allulose (or other powdered sweeteners of choice - adjust the amount to taste)

Instruction

1. Puree all ingredients in a blender, until smooth. Adjust sweetener to taste as needed.

Nutrition Per Servings: Kcal: 106, Protein: 1g, Fat: 7g, Net Carb: 6g

Keto smoked salmon and avocado plate

Prep. Time: 05 min

Cook Time: 00 min

Servings: 2 People

Ingredients

- 7 oz. smoked salmon
- 2 avocados
- ½ cup mayonnaise
- salt and pepper

Instruction

1. Split the avocado in half, remove the pit, and scoop out avocado pieces with a spoon. Place on a plate.
2. Add salmon and a hearty dollop of mayonnaise to the plate.
3. Top with freshly ground black pepper and a sprinkle of sea salt.

Nutrition Per Servings: Kcal: 811, Protein: 23g, Fat: 75g, Net Carb: 04g

Green Keto Smoothie

Prep. Time: 05 min

Cook Time: 00 min

Servings: 2 People

Ingredients

- 1 oz. kale leaves
- 1/2 avocado (peeled and stone removed)
- One stick celery (chopped)
- 2 oz. cucumber (peeled)

- 1 cup unsweetened almond milk (or regular milk)
- 1 tbsp. peanut butter (you can use any nut butter you like)
- 2 tbsp. freshly squeeze lemon juice

Instruction

1. Add all of the ingredients to a high-speed blender.
2. Pulse to combine, stopping to scrape down the sides if necessary.
3. Serve immediately garnished with fresh mint or store in the fridge for later that day.

Nutrition Per Servings: Kcal: 141, Protein: 4g, Fat: 10g, Net Carb: 4g

Broccoli Bacon Salad

Prep. Time: 10 min

Cook Time: 30 min

Servings: 6 People

Ingredients

- 1 lb (454 g) broccoli florets
- 4 small red onions or 2 large ones, sliced
- 20 slices of bacon, chopped into small pieces
- 1 cup (240 ml) coconut milk
- Salt to taste

Instruction

1. Cook the bacon first, and then cook the onions in the bacon fat.
2. Blanche the broccoli florets (or you can use them raw or soften them by boiling them first).
3. Toss the bacon pieces, onions, and broccoli florets together with the coconut milk and salt to taste. Serve at room temperature.

Nutrition Per Servings: Kcal: 280, Protein: 07g, Fat: 26g, Net Carb: 05g

Chicken Nuggets

Prep. Time: 10 min

Cook Time: 15 min

Servings: 2 People

Ingredients

- 2 chicken breasts, cut into cubes
- 1/2 cup (56 g) coconut flour
- 1 egg
- 2 Tablespoons (20 g) garlic powder
- 1 teaspoon (5 g) salt (or to taste)
- 1/4-1/2 cup (60-120 ml) ghee for shallow frying

Instruction

1. Cube the chicken breasts if you haven't done so already.
2. In a bowl, mix together the coconut flour, garlic powder, and salt. Taste the mixture to see if you'd like more salt.
3. In a separate bowl, whisk 1 egg to make the egg wash.
4. Place the ghee in a saucepan on medium heat (or use a deep fryer).
5. Dip the cubed chicken in the egg wash and then drop into the coconut flour mixture to coat it with the "breading."
6. Carefully place some of the "breaded" chicken cubes into the ghee and fry until golden (approx. 10 minutes). Make sure there's only a single layer of chicken in the pan so that they can all cook in the oil. Turn the chicken pieces to make sure they get cooked uniformly. Depending on the size of the pan, you might need to do this step in batches.
7. Place the cooked chicken pieces onto paper towels to soak up any excess oil.

Nutrition Per Servings: Kcal: 550, Protein: 60g, Fat: 27g, Net Carb: 08g

Peanut Butter Smoothie

Prep. Time: 05 min

Cook Time: 00 min

Servings: 2 People

Ingredients

- 1 cup Unsweetened Almond Milk
- Two tablespoons Peanut butter no added sugar, no added oil
- Three tablespoons Erythritol erythritol or xylitol or monk fruit
- 1/4 cup heavy cream or canned coconut cream if dairy-free
- 1 cup crushed ice or more for a frothy/ice smoothie
- One tablespoon unsweetened cocoa powder

Instruction

1. In a blender add all the ingredients, the order doesn't matter.

Blend on high speed until smooth. If you want a frothier/icy smoothie to add a few more ice cubes, blend again until smooth.

Nutrition Per Servings: Kcal: 172, Protein: 05g, Fat: 15g, Net Carb: 4g

Keto salmon-filled avocados

Prep. Time: 05 min

Cook Time: 00 min

Servings: 2 People

Ingredients

- 2 avocados
- 6 oz. smoked salmon
- ¾ cup crème fraîche or sour cream or mayonnaise
- salt and pepper

Instruction

1. Cut avocados in half and remove the pit.
2. Place a dollop of crème fraiche or mayonnaise in the hollow of the avocado and add smoked salmon on top.
3. Season to taste with salt and a squeeze lemon juice for extra flavor (and to keep the avocado from turning brown).

Nutrition Per Servings: Kcal: 717, Protein: 22g, Fat: 65g, Net Carb: 6g

Keto salmon and spinach plate

Prep. Time: 05 min

Cook Time: 10 min

Servings: 2 People

Ingredients

- 12 oz. salmon, boneless fillets, in portion pieces
- 2 tbsp butter for frying
- 3 oz. room tempered butter, for serving
- ½ red bell pepper
- 2 oz. baby spinach
- salt and pepper

Instruction

1. Fry the salmon in butter over medium heat, a few minutes on each side. Lower the heat towards the end. Season with salt and pepper.
2. Put the salmon, butter and vegetables on a plate and serve.

Nutrition Per Servings: Kcal: 791, Protein: 37g, Fat: 70g, Net Carb: 2g

Keto Flu Smoothie

Prep. Time: 05 min

Cook Time: 00 min

Servings: 1 People

Ingredients

- 1/2 cup Kale
- Two large Strawberries
- 50 grams of Avocado
- 1/2 cup Cucumber, with peel
- 1/2 cup Unsweetened Almond Milk
- 1 tsp Stevia
- 1 tsp Vanilla Extract
- 1/2 tsp Pink Himalayan Salt

Instruction

1. Add all ingredients to a blender. Blend until smooth. Chill or pour over ice.

Nutrition Per Servings: Kcal: 141, Protein: 2g, Fat: 11g, Net Carb: 7g

Chicken Bacon Burgers

Prep. Time: 10 min

Cook Time: 15 min

Servings: 8 People

Ingredients

- 4 chicken breasts
- 4 slices of bacon
- 1/4 medium onion
- 2 cloves of garlic
- 1/4 cup (60 ml) avocado oil, to cook with

Instruction

1. Food process the chicken, bacon, onion and garlic and form 8 patties. You might need to do this in batches.
2. Fry patties in the avocado oil in batches. Make sure burgers are fully cooked.
3. Serve with guacamole

Nutrition Per Servings: Kcal: 319, Protein: 25g, Fat: 24g, Net Carb: 1g

Keto Smoothie Recipe

Prep. Time: 05 min

Cook Time: 00 min

Servings: 2 People

Ingredients

- 1 1/4 cups Thai Kitchen Coconut Milk
- 1 tsp low-carb sweetener — or more
- 1/4 avocado

- 1/2 cup blackberries
- 1 tsp chia seeds
- 2 tsp unsweetened cocoa powder
- 1 tsp peanut or almond butter

Instruction

1. Add all ingredients to a blender. Blend until smooth. Chill or pour over ice.

Nutrition Per Servings: Kcal: 353, Protein: 4g, Fat: 36g, Net Carb: 7g

Basil Chicken Saute

Prep. Time: 10 min

Cook Time: 15 min

Servings: 2 People

Ingredients

- 1 chicken breast (0.5 lb or 225 g), minced or chopped very small
- 2 cloves of garlic, minced
- 1 chili pepper, diced (optional)
- 1 cup (1 large bunch) basil leaves, finely chopped
- 1 Tablespoon (15 ml) tamari sauce
- 2 Tablespoons (30 ml) avocado or coconut oil to cook in
  Salt, to taste

Instruction

1. Add oil to a frying pan and saute the garlic and pepper.
2. Then add in the minced chicken and saute until the chicken is cooked.
3. Add the tamari sauce and salt to taste. Add in the basil leaves and mix it in.

Nutrition Per Servings: Kcal: 322, Protein: 23g, Fat: 24g, Net Carb: 2g

Crispy Chicken Drumsticks

Prep. Time: 05 min

Cook Time: 40 min

Servings: 2 People

Ingredients

- 10 chicken drumsticks
- 1-2 (15-30 g) Tablespoons salt
- 3 Tablespoons (24 g) curry powder (or onion powder)
- 3 Tablespoons (30 g) garlic powder
- 1/2 Tablespoon (7 ml) of coconut oil for greasing baking tray (optional)

Instruction

1. Preheat oven to 450 F (230 C). Grease a large baking tray with coconut oil.
2. Mix the salt and spices together in a bowl.
3. Coat each drumstick with the mixture, place on the baking tray, and bake for 40 minutes.

Nutrition Per Servings: Kcal: 630, Protein: 72g, Fat: 29g, Net Carb: 4g

Keto Avocado Brownies

Prep. Time: 05 min

Cook Time: 30 min

Servings: 9 People

Ingredients

- 4 organic eggs, large 2 avocados, ripe
- 18 packets Stevia or 2/3 cup coconut sugar 2 tsp. baking soda
- 2/3 cup cocoa powder, unsweetened 6 tbsp. unsweetened
- peanut butter 1 stick (½ cup) butter, melted
- 2 tsp. pure vanilla extracts Flaky sea salt, optional
  ½ tsp. kosher salt

Instruction

1. Line a standard-sized square pan, preferably 8x8" with the parchment paper and then, preheat oven to 350 F in advance. Combine the entire ingredients (except flaky sea salt) together in a high power blended & blend on high settings until completely smooth.
2. Transfer the batter to prepared baking pan & smooth the top using a large spatula. If desired, feel free to top with the flaky sea salt.

3. Bake in the preheated oven for 20 to 25 minutes, until brownies are soft but still somewhat wet to the touch. Let cool for half an hour; slice into desired squares & serve.

Nutrition Per Servings: Kcal: 321, Protein: 08g, Fat: 29g, Net Carb: 12g

Keto mackerel and egg plate

Prep. Time: 05 min

Cook Time: 10 min

Servings: 2 People

Ingredients

- 4 eggs
- 2 tbsp butter for frying
- 8 oz. canned mackerel in tomato sauce
- 2 oz. lettuce
- ½ red onion
- ¼ cup olive oil
  salt and pepper

Instruction

1. Fry the eggs in butter, just the way you want them – sunny side up or over easy.
2. Put lettuce, thin slices of red onion and mackerel on a plate together with the eggs. Season to taste with salt and pepper. Drizzle olive oil over the salad and serve.

Nutrition Per Servings: Kcal: 689, Protein: 35g, Fat: 60g, Net Carb: 4g

Keto fried salmon with green beans

Prep. Time: 05 min

Cook Time: 10 min

Servings: 2 People

Ingredients

- 9 oz. fresh green beans
- 3 oz. butter

- 12 oz. salmon, boneless fillets in portion pieces
- ½ lemon, juice
- salt and pepper

Instruction

1. Rinse and trim the green beans.
2. Heat up the butter in a frying pan large enough to fit both the fish and vegetables.
3. Fry the green beans together with the salmon over medium heat for about 3-4 minutes on each side. Season with salt and pepper.
4. Squeeze the lemon juice over the fish and green beans in the skillet towards the end. Stir the beans every now and then.

Nutrition Per Servings: Kcal: 705, Protein: 38g, Fat: 58g, Net Carb: 6g

Guacamole Burgers

Prep. Time: 10 min

Cook Time: 20 min

Servings: 4 People

Ingredients

- 1-1.5 lbs (454-731 g) ground beef
- 4 eggs
- Coconut oil to cook with
- 1 cup (220 g) guacamole

Instruction

1. With your hands, mold the ground beef into 4 patties.
2. Cook the 4 burger patties, either in a skillet with a bit of coconut oil or on a grill.
3. Once the burgers are cooked through, place to the side.
4. Fry the eggs (preferably in coconut oil) in a skillet.
5. Place 1 fried egg on top of each burger and then top with guacamole.

Nutrition Per Servings: Kcal: 601, Protein: 44g, Fat: 45g, Net Carb: 3g

Easy Broccoli Beef Stir-Fry

Prep. Time: 10 min

Cook Time: 15 min

Servings: 2 People

Ingredients

- 2 cups (225 g) broccoli florets
- 1/2 lb (225 g) beef, sliced thin and precooked (you can use leftover Slow Cooker Asian Pot Roast (see page 70 for recipe))
- 3 cloves of garlic, minced
- 1 teaspoon (1 g) fresh ginger, grated
- 2 Tablespoons (30 ml) tamari sauce or to taste
- Avocado oil to cook in

Instruction

1. Place 2 Tablespoons of avocado oil into a skillet or saucepan on medium heat. Add the broccoli florets into the skillet.
2. When the broccoli softens to the amount you want (I like it soft, but some people like it crunchier), add in the beef slices.
3. Saute for 2 minutes and then add in the garlic, ginger, and tamari sauce.
4. Serve immediately.

Nutrition Per Servings: Kcal: 400, Protein: 22g, Fat: 30g, Net Carb: 6g

Keto fried salmon with broccoli

Prep. Time: 10 min

Cook Time: 15 min

Servings: 4 People

Ingredients

Lemon mayo
- 1 cup mayonnaise
- 2 tbsp lemon juice
Salmon with broccoli
- 1 lb broccoli
- 1¾ lbs salmon, boneless fillets

- 2 oz. butter, divided
salt and pepper

Instruction

1. Mix mayonnaise and lemon juice. Set aside for later.
2. Divide the salmon into serving-sized pieces. Season with salt and pepper.
3. Rinse and trim the broccoli, including the stem. Chop into bite-sized pieces.
4. Fry the salmon in half the butter over medium heat for a couple of minutes on each side. Lower the heat towards the end. Remove from pan and keep warm.
5. Add the remaining butter to the same skillet and cook the broccoli over medium heat for 3-4 minutes or until it is slightly softened and golden brown. Season with salt and pepper to taste.
6. Serve the fried salmon and broccoli together with a hearty dollop of lemon mayo.

Nutrition Per Servings: Kcal: 926, Protein: 44g, Fat: 80g, Net Carb: 5g

Keto fried salmon with asparagus

Prep. Time: 05 min

Cook Time: 10 min

Servings: 2 People

Ingredients

- 8 oz. green asparagus
- 3 oz. butter
- 9 oz. salmon, boneless fillets, in pieces
- salt and pepper

Instruction

1. Rinse and trim the asparagus.
2. Heat up a hearty dollop of butter in a frying pan where you can fit both the fish and vegetables.
3. Fry the asparagus over medium heat for 3-4 minutes. Season with salt and pepper. Gather everything in one half of the frying pan.
4. If necessary, add more butter and fry the pieces of salmon for a couple of minutes on each side. Stir the asparagus every now and then. Lower the heat towards the end.
5. Season the salmon and serve with the remaining butter.

Nutrition Per Servings: Kcal: 591, Protein: 28g, Fat: 52g, Net Carb: 2g

Tip!

This keto dish can be cooked with other low-carb vegetables such as zucchini, cauliflower, broccoli or spinach. Feel free to use your favorite spices to give this dish more flavor—chili powder, paprika, onion powder, some herbs, or even freshly chopped garlic and basil.

Keto baked salmon with lemon and butter

Prep. Time: 05 min

Cook Time: 10 min

Servings: 2 People

Ingredients

- 1 tbsp olive oil
- 2 lbs salmon, boneless fillets
- 1 tsp sea salt
- ground black pepper
- 7 oz. butter
- 1 lemon

Instruction

1. Preheat the oven to 400°F (200°C).
2. Grease a large baking dish with olive oil. Place the salmon, with the skin-side down, in the prepared baking dish. Generously season with salt and pepper.
3. Slice the lemon thinly and place on top of the salmon. Cover with half of the butter in thin slices.
4. Bake on middle rack for about 20–30 minutes, or until the salmon is opaque and flakes easily with a fork.
5. Heat the rest of the butter in a small sauce pan until it starts to bubble. Remove from heat and let cool a little. Gently add some lemon juice.
6. Serve with lemon butter and a side dish of your choice. See below for suggestions.

Nutrition Per Servings: Kcal: 573, Protein: 31g, Fat: 49g, Net Carb: 1g

Pan-Fried Pork Tenderloin

Prep. Time: 05 min

Cook Time: 25 min

Servings: 2 People

Ingredients

- 1 lb (454 g) pork tenderloin
- Salt and pepper to taste
- 1 Tablespoon (15 ml) coconut oil to cook in

Instruction

1. Cut the 1 lb pork tenderloin in half (to create 2 equal shorter halves).
2. Place the 1 Tablespoon of coconut oil into a frying pan on a medium heat.
3. Place the 2 pork tenderloin pieces into the pan.
4. Leave the pork to cook on its side. Sprinkle salt and pepper to taste. Once that side is cooked, turn using tongs to cook the other sides. Keep turning and cooking until the pork looks cooked on all sides.
5. Cook all sides of the pork until the meat thermometer shows an internal temperature of just below 145 F (63 C). The pork will keep on cooking a bit after you take it out of the pan.
6. Let the pork sit for a few minutes and then slice into 1-inch thick slices with a sharp knife.

Nutrition Per Servings: Kcal: 332, Protein: 45g, Fat: 15g, Net Carb: 0g

Rosemary Baked Salmon

Prep. Time: 05 min

Cook Time: 30 min

Servings: 2 People

Ingredients

- 2 salmon filets (fresh or defrosted)
- 1 Tablespoon (2 g) fresh rosemary leaves
- 1/4 cup (60 ml) olive oil
- 1 teaspoon (5 g) salt (optional or to taste)

Instruction

1. Preheat oven to 350 F (175 C).
2. Mix the olive oil, rosemary, and salt together in a bowl.
3. Place one salmon filet at a time into the mixture and rub mixture onto the filet.
4. Wrap each filet in a piece of aluminum foil with some of the remaining mixture.
5. Bake for 25-30 minutes.

Nutrition Per Servings: Kcal: 432, Protein: 63g, Fat: 18g, Net Carb: 0g

Keto ground beef and green beans

Prep. Time: 05 min

Cook Time: 15 min

Servings: 2 People

Ingredients

- 12 oz. ground beef
- 9 oz. fresh green beans
- 3½ oz. butter
- salt and pepper
- 1/3 cup mayonnaise (optional)

Instruction

1. Rinse and trim the green beans.
2. Heat up a generous dollop of butter in a frying pan where you can fit both the ground beef and the green beans.
3. Brown the ground beef on high heat until it's almost done. Add salt and pepper.
4. Lower the heat somewhat. Add more butter and fry the beans for 5 minutes in the same pan. Stir the ground beef every now and then.
5. Season beans with salt and pepper. Serve with remaining butter and add mayonnaise or crème fraiche if you need more fat for satiety.

Nutrition Per Servings: Kcal: 735, Protein: 36g, Fat: 62g, Net Carb: 5g

Keto ground beef and broccoli

Prep. Time: 05 min

Cook Time: 15 min

Servings: 2 People

Ingredients

- 2/3 lb ground beef
- 3 oz. butter
- ½ lb broccoli
- salt and pepper
- ½ cup mayonnaise (optional)

Instruction

1. Rinse and trim the broccoli, including the stem. Cut into small florets. Peel the stem and cut into small pieces.
2. Heat up a hearty dollop of butter in a frying pan where you can fit both the ground beef and broccoli.
3. Brown the ground beef on high heat until it is almost done. Season to taste with salt and pepper.
4. Lower the heat, add more butter and fry the broccoli for 3-5 minutes. Stir the ground beef every now and then.
5. Season the broccoli. Top with the remaining butter and serve while still hot. It's also delicious to serve with an extra dollop of crème fraiche or mayonnaise.

Nutrition Per Servings: Kcal: 646, Protein: 33g, Fat: 55g, Net Carb: 5g

Keto turkey plate

Prep. Time: 05 min

Cook Time: 00 min

Servings: 2 People

Ingredients

- 6 oz. deli turkey
- 1 avocado, sliced
- 2 oz. lettuce
- 3 oz. cream cheese

- 4 tbsp olive oil
  salt and pepper

Instruction

1. Divide the ingredients relevant to the serving number and place an equal amount of turkey, avocado, lettuce, and cream cheese on each plate.
2. Drizzle olive oil over the vegetables and season to taste with salt and pepper.

Nutrition Per Servings: Kcal: 650, Protein: 22g, Fat: 59g, Net Carb: 7g

Tip!

Feel free to add a couple of sticks of celery, and fill the groove in the celery with the cream cheese. Crunch!

Always check the ingredients on deli meats before purchasing them, they can vary significantly. Ask the staff at your local delicatessen for advice.

Cucumber Ginger Shrimp

Prep. Time: 05 min

Cook Time: 10 min

Servings: 1 People

Ingredients

- 1 large cucumber, peeled and sliced into 1/2-inch round slices
- 10-15 large shrimp/prawns (defrosted if frozen)
- 1 teaspoon (1 g) fresh ginger, grated
- Salt to taste
- Coconut oil to cook with

Instruction

1. Place 1 Tablespoon (15 ml) of coconut oil into a frying pan on medium heat.
2. Add in the ginger and the cucumber and sauté for 2-3 minutes.
3. Add in the shrimp and cook until they turn pink and are no longer translucent.
4. Add salt to taste and serve.

Nutrition Per Servings: Kcal: 250, Protein: 20g, Fat: 16g, Net Carb: 4g

Dinners Recipes

Keto Cream Cheese Pancake

Prep. Time: 05 min

Cook Time: 10 min

Servings: 1 People

Ingredients

- 2 eggs
- 2 oz. cream cheese
- 1 tbsp coconut flour
- ½ tsp cinnamon
- 1 packet stevia

Instruction

1. Beat or blend together the ingredients until the batter is smooth and free of lumps.
2. Two pancakes is equivalent to one serving. On medium-high, heat up a non-stick skillet or pan with coconut oil or salted butter.
3. Ladle the batter on to the pan. Heat until bubbles begin to form on top. Flip over, and cook until the other side is sufficiently browned.
4. Serve. Top with sugar-free maple syrup and grass-fed butter.

Nutrition Per Servings: Kcal: 299, Protein: 16g, Fat: 25g, Net Carb: 3g

Keto oven-baked chicken in garlic butter

Prep. Time: 10 min

Cook Time: 55 min

Servings: 4 People

Ingredients

- 3 lbs chicken, a whole bird
- 2 tsp sea salt
- ½ tsp ground black pepper
- 6 oz. butter

- 2 garlic cloves, minced

Instruction

1. Preheat the oven to 400°F (200°C). Season the chicken with salt and pepper, both inside and out.
2. Place chicken breast up in a baking dish.
3. Combine the garlic and butter in a small saucepan over medium heat. The butter should not turn brown, just melt.
4. Let the butter cool for a couple of minutes.
5. Pour the garlic butter over and inside the chicken. Bake on lower oven rack for 1-1 ½ hours, or until internal temperature reaches 180°F (82°C). Baste with the juices from the bottom of the pan every 20 minutes.
6. Serve with the juices and a side dish of your choice.

Nutrition Per Servings: Kcal: 1035, Protein: 59g, Fat: 87g, Net Carb: 1g

Keto fried chicken with cabbage

Prep. Time: 05 min

Cook Time: 15 min

Servings: 2 People

Ingredients

- 12 oz. green cabbage
- 3½ oz. butter
- 10 oz. boneless chicken thighs
- salt and pepper

Instruction

1. Shred the cabbage finely using a sharp knife or a food processor.
2. Heat up a generous dollop of butter in a frying pan large enough to fit both the chicken and the cabbage.
3. Season the chicken. Fry over medium heat for about 4 minutes on each side or until golden brown and fully cooked through.
4. Add more butter and add the cabbage to the same pan. Fry for another 5 minutes.
5. Season the cabbage and serve with the remaining butter.

Nutrition Per Servings: Kcal: 774, Protein: 27g, Fat: 66g, Net Carb: 6g

Turkey Arugula Salad

Prep. Time: 05 min

Cook Time: 00 min

Servings: 2 People

Ingredients

- oz (100 g) arugula leaves
- 4 oz (115 g) turkey deli meat or turkey breast meat, diced
- 10 raspberries (or blueberries)
- 1 cucumber, peeled and diced
- 2 Tablespoons (30 ml) olive oil
- Juice from 1/2 a lime

Instruction

1. Toss all the ingredients together in a large bowl and enjoy.

Nutrition Per Servings: Kcal: 260, Protein: 20g, Fat: 15g, Net Carb: 6g

Keto fried chicken with broccoli and butter

Prep. Time: 10 min

Cook Time: 25 min

Servings: 4 People

Ingredients

- 5 oz. butter, divided
- 1½ lbs boneless chicken thighs
- salt and pepper
- 1 lb broccoli
- ½ leek
- 1 tsp garlic powder

Instruction

1. Melt half of the butter in a large frying pan, over medium high heat.
2. Generously season the chicken with salt and pepper and then add it to the pan, flipping the chicken until browned on both sides, for approximately 20-25 minutes

(depending upon the size of the chicken thighs.) Remove from pan, and keep warm under aluminum foil or on low heat in the oven.

3. While the chicken is cooking, rinse and trim the broccoli, including the stem. Chop into bite-sized pieces. Rinse the leek, being careful to remove sandy deposits between layers. Coarsely chop the leek.

4. In a separate skillet, melt the remaining butter over medium heat, mixing in the garlic powder, salt and pepper. Add the leek to the pan, stirring until it starts to soften, and then add the broccoli. Cook for a few minutes, until the broccoli becomes slightly tender.

5. Serve the chicken and vegetables with an extra dollop of butter melting on top.

Nutrition Per Servings: Kcal: 774, Protein: 27g, Fat: 66g, Net Carb: 6g

Tip!

Switch up the flavors of this workhorse dish with different seasonings (like curry, paprika, or dried herbs) for the chicken. Or try one of our compound butters on top. Alternatively, you can mix things up by switching to a dip; mayo with a dash of Sriracha sauce tastes great and gives the dish a real kick!

Cumin Crusted Lamb Chops

Prep. Time: 15 min

Cook Time: 15 min

Servings: 4 People

Ingredients

- 2 racks of lamb (3 lb or 1.3 kg)
- ¾ cup (72 g) cumin powder
- 3 Tablespoons (18 g) paprika
- 1 teaspoon (1 g) chili powder (more if preferred)
- 1 Tablespoon (15 g) salt (less if preferred)

Instruction

1. Cut the racks of lamb into individual lamb chops (approx 20 chops).
2. Combine the spices and salt and dip the lamb chops into it.
3. Grill the lamb until done to the level you enjoy.

Nutrition Per Servings: Kcal: 702, Protein: 47g, Fat: 60g, Net Carb: 2g

Nut Free Keto Brownie

Prep. Time: 10 min

Cook Time: 20 min

Servings: 12 People

Ingredients

- 6 medium eggs
- 1 to 2 tbsp. unsweetened cocoa
- 3 to 4 tbsp. melted butter
- 1 cup softened cream cheese 2 tsp. vanilla
- ½ tsp. baking powder
- 4 tbsp. granulated sweetener, any of your choice or to taste

Instruction

1. Put the entire ingredients together in a large-sized mixing bowl & blend using a stick blender with the blade attachment until completely smooth.
2. Pour the prepared mixture into a lined square baking dish (preferably 8 ½").
3. Bake until cooked on the middle, for 20 to 25 minutes, at 350F.
4. Slice into your favorite shapes such as rectangle, squares, bars or triangle wedges.

Nutrition Per Servings: Kcal: 140, Protein: 14g, Fat: 105g, Net Carb: 2g

Keto chicken pesto

Prep. Time: 10 min

Cook Time: 15 min

Servings: 4 People

Ingredients

- 11/3 lbs boneless chicken thighs
- 1/3 cup sugar-free green pesto
- 5 oz. cherry tomatoes, halved
- 4 oz. feta cheese, crumbled or cubed
- 12 oz. zucchini or zucchini noodles
- 3 tbsp olive oil

Instruction

1. Place the chicken thighs in a medium pot and add cold water until the chicken is just covered.
2. Bring to a boil. Then reduce the heat to medium-low and simmer for 15 minutes or until the chicken is thoroughly cooked.
3. Remove the chicken from the water and shred it using two forks. Set aside.
4. Spiralize the zucchini and place the zoodles in a large mixing bowl.
5. Pour the pesto over the zoodles, and toss with tongs to completely coat the zoodles.
6. Add shredded chicken breast, tomatoes, and feta to the zoodles and gently toss with tongs until evenly combined. Drizzle with olive oil.

Nutrition Per Servings: Kcal: 616, Protein: 32g, Fat: 51g, Net Carb: 5g

Cheese, Mortadella and Salami

Prep. Time: 5 min

Cook Time: 5 min

Servings: 4 People

Ingredients

- 10 slices Provolone cheese
- 4 ounces of mayonnaise
- 10 slices Mortadella
- 10 slices Genoa salami
- 10 pitted olives

Instruction

1. Add a thin layer of mayonnaise onto each slice of cheese, then add another layer of Mortadella on top of the mayonnaise.
2. Top up with a slice of Genoa salami, roll them up, and place olives on the top.
3. For a party of 10, this is a great way to cut costs.

Nutrition Per Servings: Kcal: 381, Protein: 17g, Fat: 32g, Net Carb: 5g

Keto chicken and green beans plate

Prep. Time: 5 min

Cook Time: 10 min

Servings: 2 People

Ingredients

- 7 oz. fresh green beans
- 2 tbsp butter for frying
- 1 lb of cooked chicken
- 4 oz. butter for serving
- salt and pepper

Instruction

1. Fry the green beans in butter over medium heat for a couple of minutes. Season with salt and pepper to taste.
2. Put chicken, green beans and butter on a plate and serve.

Nutrition Per Servings: Kcal: 896, Protein: 75g, Fat: 65g, Net Carb: 2g

Tips

We've used rotisserie chicken for this plate but feel free cook the chicken from scratch if you prefer. Here's a simple recipe. Always make sure that poultry is fully cooked (internal temperature of at least 165°F (74°C) before serving.

Keto chicken and Feta cheese plate

Prep. Time: 5 min

Cook Time: 00 min

Servings: 2 People

Ingredients

- 1 lb of rotisserie chicken
- 7 oz. feta cheese
- 2 tomatoes
- 2 cups leafy greens

- 10 black olives
- 1/3 cup olive oil
- salt and pepper

Instruction

1. Slice the tomatoes and put them on a plate together with chicken, feta cheese, lettuce and olives.
2. Season with salt and pepper to taste. Serve with olive oil.

Nutrition Per Servings: Kcal: 1200, Protein: 63g, Fat: 100g, Net Carb: 100g

Tip!

We've used rotisserie chicken for this plate but feel free cook the chicken from scratch if you prefer. Always make sure that poultry is fully cooked (internal temperature of at least 165°F) before serving.

Keto chicken and cabbage plate

Prep. Time: 5 min

Cook Time: 00 min

Servings: 2 People

Ingredients

- 1 lb of rotisserie chicken
- 7 oz. fresh green cabbage
- ½ red onion
- 1 tbsp olive oil
- ½ cup mayonnaise
- salt and pepper

Instruction

1. Shred the cabbage using a sharp knife or a mandolin and place it on a plate.
2. Slice the onion thinly and add it to the plate, together with the rotisserie chicken and a hearty dollop of mayonnaise.
3. Drizzle olive oil over the cabbage and add some salt and pepper to taste.

Nutrition Per Servings: Kcal: 1041, Protein: 48g, Fat: 90g, Net Carb: 7g

Tip!

For this dish we've used rotisserie chicken but you can use any kind of leftover chicken. Or, pan-fry a piece or two of raw chicken if you wish. Just make sure it's fully cooked through (internal temperature of 165°F) before serving.

Mushroom brunch

Prep. Time: 05 min

Cook Time: 15 min

Servings: 4 People

Ingredients

- 250g mushrooms
- 1 garlic clove
- 1 tbsp olive oil
- 160g bag kale
- 4 eggs

Instruction

1. Slice the mushrooms and crush the garlic clove. Heat the olive oil in a large non-stick frying pan, then fry the garlic over a low heat for 1 min. Add the mushrooms and cook until soft. Then, add the kale. If the kale won't all fit in the pan, add half and stir until wilted, then add the rest. Once all the kale is wilted, season.
2. Now crack in the eggs and keep them cooking gently for 2-3 mins. Then, cover with the lid to for a further 2-3 mins or until the eggs are cooked to your liking. Serve with bread.

Nutrition Per Servings: Kcal: 154, Protein: 13g, Fat: 11g, Net Carb: 01g

Herb omelette with fried tomatoes

Prep. Time: 05 min

Cook Time: 05 min

Servings: 2 People

Ingredients

- 1 tsp rapeseed oil
- 3 tomatoes , halved
- 4 large eggs
- 1 tbsp chopped parsley
- 1 tbsp chopped basil

Instruction

1. Heat the oil in a small non-stick frying pan, then cook the tomatoes cut-side down until starting to soften and colour. Meanwhile, beat the eggs with the herbs and plenty of freshly ground black pepper in a small bowl.
2. Scoop the tomatoes from the pan and put them on two serving plates. Pour the egg mixture into the pan and stir gently with a wooden spoon so the egg that sets on the base of the pan moves to enable uncooked egg to flow into the space. Stop stirring when it's nearly cooked to allow it to set into an omelette. Cut into four and serve with the tomatoes.

Nutrition Per Servings: Kcal: 204, Protein: 17g, Fat: 13g, Net Carb: 04g

Egg with Bacon & Asparagus Soldiers

Prep. Time: 05 min

Cook Time: 30 min

Servings: 4 People

Ingredients

- 8 asparagus spears (about 300g), woody ends discarded
- 4 long thin slices rustic bread (preferably sourdough)
- 8 rashers smoked streaky bacon or pancetta
- 4 duck eggs

Instruction

1. Heat your grill to high. Snap off the woody ends of the asparagus spears and discard. Cut the bread into 12 soldiers, a little shorter than the asparagus.
2. Place a spear onto each soldier and wrap tightly with a rasher of bacon. Place on a baking tray, season and grill for 15 mins or until the bacon is crisp.

3. Bring a pan of salted water to the boil and simmer the duck eggs for about 7 mins, to get a runny yolk and a cooked white. Serve immediately with the warm soldiers for dipping.

Nutrition Per Servings: Kcal: 306, Protein: 20g, Fat: 19g, Net Carb: 14g

Soft-boiled eggs with pancetta avocado

Prep. Time: 05 min

Cook Time: 10 min

Servings: 2 People

Ingredients

- 4 eggs
- 1 tbsp vegetable oil
- 1 ripe avocado , cut into slices
- 100g smoked pancetta rashers

Instruction

1. Bring a large saucepan of salted water to the boil. Carefully drop the eggs into the water and boil for 5 mins for runny yolks.
2. Meanwhile, heat the oil in a non-stick pan and wrap each avocado slice in pancetta. Fry for 2-3 mins over a high heat until cooked and crisp.
3. Serve the eggs in egg cups with the pancetta avocado soldiers on the side for dipping.

Nutrition Per Servings: Kcal: 517, Protein: 22g, Fat: 46g, Net Carb: 01g

Gordon's eggs Benedict

Prep. Time: 05 min

Cook Time: 20 min

Servings: 2 People

Ingredients

- 3 tbsp white wine vinegar

- 4 large free range eggs
- 2 toasting muffins
- 1 batch hot hollandaise sauce (see 'Goes well with' below)
- 4 slices Parma ham (or Serrano or Bayonne)

Instruction

1. Bring a deep saucepan of water to the boil (at least 2 litres) and add 3 tbsp white wine vinegar. Break the eggs into 4 separate coffee cups or ramekins. Split the muffins, toast them and warm some plates.
2. Swirl the vinegared water briskly to form a vortex and slide in an egg. It will curl round and set to a neat round shape. Cook for 2-3 mins, then remove with a slotted spoon.
3. Repeat with the other eggs, one at a time, re-swirling the water as you slide in the eggs. Spread some sauce on each muffin, scrunch a slice of ham on top, then top with an egg. Spoon over the remaining hollandaise and serve at once.

Nutrition Per Servings: Kcal: 705, Protein: 18g, Fat: 64g, Net Carb: 16g

Lamb & lettuce pan-fry

Prep. Time: 05 min

Cook Time: 15 min

Servings: 4 People

Ingredients

- 25g butter
- 4 lamb neck fillets, cut into chunks
- 2 handfuls frozen peas
- 150ml chicken stock
- 3 Baby Gem lettuces , cut into quarters

Instruction

1. Heat the butter in a frying pan until sizzling, then add the lamb. Season with salt, if you like, and pepper, then cook for 6-7 mins until browned on all sides. Scatter in the peas, pour in the stock, then bring up to a simmer and gently cook until the peas have defrosted.
2. Add the lettuce to the pan and simmer for a few mins until just starting to wilt, but still vibrant green. Serve scooped straight from the pan, with buttered new potatoes.

Nutrition Per Servings: Kcal: 465, Protein: 30g, Fat: 37g, Net Carb: 3g

Chilli avocado

Prep. Time: 02 min

Cook Time: 00 min

Servings: 1 People

Ingredients

- ½ small avocado
- ¼ tsp chilli flakes
- juice of ¼ lime

Instruction

1. Sprinkle the avocado with the chilli flakes, lime juice and a little black pepper, and eat with a spoon.

Nutrition Per Servings: Kcal: 102, Protein: 1g, Fat: 10g, Net Carb: 1g

Italian keto plate

Prep. Time: 05 min

Cook Time: 00 min

Servings: 4 People

Ingredients

- 7 oz. fresh mozzarella cheese
- 7 oz. prosciutto, sliced
- 2 tomatoes
- 1/3 cup olive oil
- 10 green olives
- salt and pepper

Instruction

1. Put tomatoes, prosciutto, cheese and olives on a plate. Serve with olive oil and season with salt and pepper to taste..

Nutrition Per Servings: Kcal: 824, Protein: 38g, Fat: 65g, Net Carb: 10g

Keto fried salmon with broccoli and cheese

Prep. Time: 05 min

Cook Time: 00 min

Servings: 4 People

Ingredients

- 1 lb broccoli
- 3 oz. butter
- salt and pepper
- 5 oz. grated cheddar cheese
- 1½ lbs salmon
- 1 lime (optional)

Instruction

1. Put tomatoes, prosciutto, cheese and olives on a plate. Serve with olive oil and season with salt and pepper to taste..

Nutrition Per Servings: Kcal: 824, Protein: 38g, Fat: 65g, Net Carb: 10g

Keto Ground Beef Enchiladas

Prep. Time: 15 min

Cook Time: 06 min

Servings: 4 People

Ingredients

- 1 pound ground beef
- homemade keto taco seasoning
- 2 cups Mexican blend cheese, shredded
- 1/2 cup red enchilada sauce, warmed in microwave
- 8 teaspoons sour cream
- 2 green onions, sliced

Instruction

1. Cook ground beef in a skillet on the stove with homemade keto seasoning. Set aside.
2. Preheat oven to 350 degrees. Prepare a baking sheet pan with parchment paper or silicone mat.
3. Arrange shredded cheese into 8 separate flat circles on the sheet pan, using about 1/4 cup cheese for each one. You may have to use two sheet pans to make 8 enchilada shells.
4. Bake for about 6 minutes until cheese is bubbling and the outside of the cheese circles starts to brown.
5. While still warm and bendable, flip each cheese circle over. Roll each one with 1/2 cup ground beef, and pour warm enchilada sauce over the top.
6. Add 1 teaspoon of sour cream to each enchilada, and a few sliced onions to the tops.

Nutrition Per Servings: Kcal: 485, Protein: 29g, Fat: 38g, Net Carb: 6g

Grilled Buttermilk Chicken

Prep. Time: 10 min

Cook Time: 10 min

Servings: 4 People

Ingredients

- 1-1/2 cups buttermilk
- 4 fresh thyme sprigs
- 4 garlic cloves, halved
- 1/2 teaspoon salt
- 12 boneless skinless chicken breast halves (about 4-1/2 pounds)

Instruction

1. Place the buttermilk, thyme, garlic and salt in a large bowl or shallow dish. Add chicken and turn to coat. Refrigerate 8 hours or overnight, turning occasionally.
2. Drain chicken, discarding marinade. Grill, covered, over medium heat until a thermometer reads 165°, 5-7 minutes per side.

Nutrition Per Servings: Kcal: 190, Protein: 35g, Fat: 04g, Net Carb: 1g

Pistachio Salmon

Prep. Time: 10 min

Cook Time: 20 min

Servings: 4 People

Ingredients

- 1/3 cup pistachios, finely chopped
- 1/4 cup panko bread crumbs
- 1/4 cup grated Parmesan cheese
- 1 salmon fillet (1 pound)
- 1/2 teaspoon salt
- 1/4 teaspoon pepper

Instruction

1. Preheat oven to 400°. In a shallow bowl, toss pistachios with bread crumbs and cheese.
2. Place salmon on a greased foil-lined 15x10x1-in. pan, skin side down; sprinkle with salt and pepper. Top with pistachio mixture, pressing to adhere. Bake, uncovered, until fish just begins to flake easily with a fork, 15-20 minutes.

Nutrition Per Servings: Kcal: 270, Protein: 23g, Fat: 17g, Net Carb: 6g

Sauteed Radishes with Green Beans

Prep. Time: 10 min

Cook Time: 10 min

Servings: 4 People

Ingredients

- 1 tablespoon butter
- 1/2 pound fresh green or wax beans, trimmed
- 1 cup thinly sliced radishes
- 1/2 teaspoon sugar
- 1/4 teaspoon salt
- 2 tablespoons pine nuts, toasted

Instruction

1. In a large skillet, heat butter over medium-high heat. Add beans; cook and stir 3-4 minutes or until crisp-tender.
2. Add radishes; cook 2-3 minutes longer or until vegetables are tender, stirring occasionally. Stir in sugar and salt; sprinkle with nuts.
   Note: To toast nuts, bake in a shallow pan in a 350° oven for 5-10 minutes or cook in a skillet over low heat until lightly browned, stirring occasionally.

Nutrition Per Servings: Kcal: 75, Protein: 2g, Fat: 6g, Net Carb: 4g

Zucchini Noodles

Prep. Time: 5 min

Cook Time: 5 min

Servings: 4 People

Ingredients

- 4 large zucchini

Instruction

1. Wash the Zucchini thoroughly.
2. Cut the Zucchini noodles using a spiralizer, a mandolin slicer or a veg-
3. etable peeler.
4. Set aside on paper towels for 10 minutes.
5. Cook the Zucchini noodles by boiling them, sauté them in oil or sim-
6. mer them in a sauce

Nutrition Per Servings: Kcal: 3, Protein: 0.43g, Fat: 0.06g, Net Carb: 0.5g

Bonus Recipes

Grilled Peppered Steaks

Prep. Time: 05 min

Cook Time: 20 min

Servings: 4 People

Ingredients

- 1-1/2 to 2 teaspoons coarsely ground pepper
- 1 teaspoon onion salt
- 1 teaspoon garlic salt
- 1/4 teaspoon paprika
- 4 boneless beef top loin steaks (8 ounces each)

Instruction

1. In a small bowl, combine the pepper, onion salt, garlic salt and, if desired, paprika Rub onto both sides of steaks.
2. Grill, covered, over medium heat until meat reaches desired doneness (for medium-rare, a thermometer should read 135°; medium, 140°; medium-well, 145°), 8-10 minutes on each side.

Editor's Note

Top loin steak may be labeled as strip steak, Kansas City steak, New York strip steak, ambassador steak or boneless club steak in your region.

Nutrition Per Servings: Kcal: 301, Protein: 48g, Fat: 10g, Net Carb: 1g

Grilled Lemon-Garlic Salmon

Prep. Time: 05 min

Cook Time: 25 min

Servings: 4 People

Ingredients

- 2 garlic cloves, minced
- 2 teaspoons grated lemon zest
- 1/2 teaspoon salt

- 1/2 teaspoon minced fresh rosemary
- 1/2 teaspoon pepper
- 4 salmon fillets (6 ounces each)

Instruction

1. In a small bowl, mix the first five ingredients; rub over fillets. Let stand 15 minutes. Moisten a paper towel with cooking oil; using long-handled tongs, rub on grill rack to coat lightly.
2. Place salmon on grill rack, skin side up. Grill, covered, over medium heat or broil 4 in. from heat 4 minutes. Turn; grill 3-6 minutes longer or until fish just begins to flake easily with a fork.

Nutrition Per Servings: Kcal: 268, Protein: 29g, Fat: 16g, Net Carb: 1g

Buffalo Pulled Chicken

Prep. Time: 05 min

Cook Time: 03 h

Servings: 6 People

Ingredients

- 1/2 cup Buffalo wing sauce
- 2 tablespoons ranch salad dressing mix
- 4 boneless skinless chicken breast halves (6 ounces each)

Instruction

1. In a 3-qt. slow cooker, mix wing sauce and dressing mix. Add chicken. Cook, covered, on low until meat is tender, 3-4 hours.
2. Shred chicken with 2 forks. If desired, serve on celery, top with additional wing sauce and cheese, and serve with ranch dressing.

Nutrition Per Servings: Kcal: 147, Protein: 23g, Fat: 03g, Net Carb: 6g

Cheesy Roasted Broccoli

Prep. Time: 05 min

Cook Time: 10 min

Servings: 6 People

Ingredients

- ¼ cup ranch dressing
- 4 cups broccoli florets
- ¼ cup heavy whipping cream
- ½ cup cheddar cheese, shredded
- Salt and pepper to taste

Instruction

1. Preheat your oven to 375 degrees F.
2. Put all the ingredients in a bowl and mix.
3. Arrange the broccoli mix on a baking dish.
4. Bake in the oven for 10 minutes or until tender enough.

Nutrition Per Servings: Kcal: 80, Protein: 4g, Fat: 6g, Net Carb: 4g

Quick Garlic-Lime Chicken

Prep. Time: 10 min

Cook Time: 40 min

Servings: 6 People

Ingredients

- 1/3 cup soy sauce
- 1/4 cup fresh lime juice
- 1 tablespoon Worcestershire sauce
- 1/2 teaspoon ground mustard
- 2 garlic cloves, minced
- 6 boneless skinless chicken breast halves (6 ounces each)
- 1/2 teaspoon pepper

Instruction

1. In a shallow dish, combine the first 5 ingredients; add chicken and turn to coat. Cover and refrigerate for at least 30 minutes.
2. Drain discard marinade. Sprinkle chicken with pepper. Grill , covered, over medium heat until a thermometer reads, 165°, 7-8 minutes on each side.

Nutrition Per Servings: Kcal: 191, Protein: 35g, Fat: 04g, Net Carb: 1g

Keto Fat Bombs

Prep. Time: 30 min

Cook Time: 00 min

Servings: 10 People

Ingredients

- 8 tablespoons butter
- ¼ cup Swerve
- ½ teaspoon vanilla extract
- Salt to taste
- 2 cups almond flour
- 2/3 cup chocolate chips

Instruction

1. In a bowl, beat the butter until fluffy.
2. Stir in the sugar, salt and vanilla.
3. Mix well.
4. Add the almond flour.
5. Fold in the chocolate chips.
6. Cover the bowl with cling wrap and refrigerate for 20 minutes.
7. Create balls from the dough.

Nutrition Per Servings: Kcal: 176, Protein: 00g, Fat: 15g, Net Carb: 10g

Oven-Roasted Salmon

Prep. Time: 05 min

Cook Time: 20 min

Servings: 4 People

Ingredients

- 1 center-cut salmon fillet (1-1/2 pounds)
- 1 tablespoon olive oil
- 1/2 teaspoon salt
- 1/4 teaspoon pepper

Instruction

1. Place a large cast-iron or other ovenproof skillet in a cold oven. Preheat oven to 450°. Meanwhile, brush salmon with oil and sprinkle with salt and pepper.
2. Carefully remove skillet from oven. Place fish, skin side down, in skillet. Return to oven; bake uncovered, until salmon flakes easily and a thermometer reads 125°, 14-18 minutes. Cut salmon into four equal portions.

Nutrition Per Servings: Kcal: 291, Protein: 30g, Fat: 20g, Net Carb: 0g

Ham Pickle Pinwheels

Prep. Time: 05 min

Cook Time: 20 min

Servings: 7 People

Ingredients

- 1 package (8 ounces) cream cheese, cubed
- 1/4 pound sliced Genoa salami
- 1 tablespoon prepared horseradish
- 7 slices deli ham
- 14 to 21 okra pickles or dill pickle spears

Instruction

1. In a food processor, add the cream cheese, salami and horseradish; cover and process until blended. Spread over ham slices.

2. Remove stems and ends of okra pickles. Place 2 or 3 okra pickles or 1 dill pickle down the center of each ham slice. Roll up tightly and cover. Refrigerate for at least 2 hours. Cut into 1-in. pieces.

Test Kitchen Tips

- A pickle is actually a pickled cucumber that has been submerged and fermented in a brine or vinegar. The concept of pickles dates all the way back to 2030 BCE.
- Use deli ham or ham you've made yourself. Both are delicious!
- Check out 30 appetizers ready in 15 minutes or less.

Nutrition Per Servings: Kcal: 34, Protein: 2g, Fat: 3g, Net Carb: 1g

Coconut Crack Bars

Prep. Time: 02 min

Cook Time: 05 min

Servings: 20 People

Ingredients

- 3 cups coconut flakes (unsweetened)
- 1 cup coconut oil
- ¼ cup maple syrup

Instruction

1. Line a baking sheet with parchment paper.
2. Put coconut in a bowl.
3. Add the oil and syrup.
4. Mix well.
5. Pour the mixture into the pan.
6. Refrigerate until firm.
7. Slice into bars before serving.

Nutrition Per Servings: Kcal: 147, Protein: 0.4g, Fat: 16g, Net Carb: 3g

Lemon-Butter Tilapia with Almonds

Prep. Time: 05 min

Cook Time: 05 min

Servings: 4 People

Ingredients

- 4 tilapia fillets (4 ounces each)
- 1/2 teaspoon salt
- 1/4 teaspoon pepper
- 1 tablespoon olive oil
- 1/4 cup butter, cubed
- 1/4 cup white wine or chicken broth
- 2 tablespoons lemon juice
- 1/4 cup sliced almonds

Instruction

1. Sprinkle fillets with salt and pepper. In a large non-stick skillet, heat oil over medium heat. Add fillets; cook until fish just begins to flake easily with a fork, 2-3 minutes on each side. Remove and keep warm.
2. Add butter, wine and lemon juice to same pan; cook and stir until butter is melted. Serve with fish; sprinkle with almonds.

Nutrition Per Servings: Kcal: 270, Protein: 22g, Fat: 19g, Net Carb: 2g

Keto Pancakes

Prep. Time: 05 min

Cook Time: 10 min

Servings: 10 People

Ingredients

- ½ cup almond flour
- 4 oz. cream cheese
- 4 eggs
- 1 teaspoon lemon zest
- 1 tablespoon butter

Instruction

1. In a bowl, mix all the ingredients except the butter.
2. Mix until smooth.
3. In a pan over medium heat, put the butter and let it melt.
4. Pour three tablespoons of batter and cook for 2 minutes or until golden.
5. Flip the pancake and cook for another 2 minutes.
6. Repeat the same steps with the rest of the batter.

Nutrition Per Servings: Kcal: 84, Protein: 4g, Fat: 8g, Net Carb: 0.6g

Cream Cheese Muffins

Prep. Time: 10 min

Cook Time: 10 min

Servings: 6 People

Ingredients

- 4 tablespoons melted butter, plus more for the muffin tin
- 1 cup almond flour
- ¾ tablespoon baking powder
- 2 large eggs, lightly beaten
- 2 ounces cream cheese mixed with 2 tablespoons heavy (whipping) cream
- Handfulshredded Mexican blend cheese

Instruction

1. Preheat the oven to 400°F. Coat six cups of a muffin tin with butter.
2. In a small bowl, mix together the almond flour and baking powder.
3. In a medium bowl, mix together the eggs, cream cheese–heavy cream mixture, shredded cheese, and 4 tablespoons of the melted butter.
4. Pour the flour mixture into the egg mixture, and beat with a hand mixer until thoroughly mixed.
5. Pour the batter into the prepared muffin cups.
6. Bake for 12 minutes, or until golden brown on top, and serve.

Nutrition Per Servings: Kcal: 247, Protein: 8g, Fat: 23g, Net Carb: 6g

Keto Palmini Spaghetti Bolognese

Prep. Time: 15 min

Cook Time: 20 min

Servings: 4 People

Ingredients

- 2 cans palmini linguine noodles, drained (450 g/ 1 lb)
- 500 g ground beef (1.1 lb)
- 1 1/4 cups Homemade Marinara Sauce, 1 recipe (300 ml/ 10 fl oz)
- Optional: 4 tbsp grated Parmesan cheese or more, to serve (20 g/ 0.7 oz)
- Optional: fresh basil leaves, to serve

Instruction

1. Open the Palmini cans and drain the liquid by pouring the content of both cans in a colander.Keto Palmini Spaghetti Bolognese
2. Rinse with water and set aside. The noodles can be eaten as they are or you can place them in a pot with hot water to heat up for 30 to 60 seconds, or heat in a microwave for 30-60 seconds. If you want to warm them up, do that just before serving.
3. Meanwhile, prepare the Marinara Sauce and the beef.Keto Palmini Spaghetti Bolognese
4. Place the ground meat in a cast iron skillet or a non stick pan. (If using cast iron, add a few tablespoons of water.) Cook over a medium-high heat until browned and opaque, for about 10 minutes. Add the Marinara Sauce and cook to heat through. Take off the heat.Keto Palmini Spaghetti Bolognese
5. Place the marinara flavoured meat in a serving bowl and top with the noodles.Keto Palmini Spaghetti Bolognese
6. Optionally serve each with 1 to 2 tablespoons of grated parmesan and a few basil leaves.
7. To store, refrigerate the meat mixture for up to 4 days or freeze for up to 3 months. Palmini are best prepared fresh — it only takes a minute!

Nutrition Per Servings: Kcal: 474, Protein: 25g, Fat: 27g, Net Carb: 6g

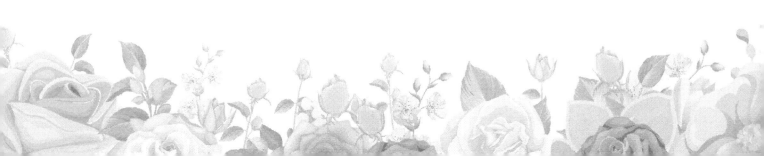

Mashed Cauliflower with Chives

Prep. Time: 15 min

Cook Time: 25 min

Servings: 4 People

Ingredients

- 2 cups chicken broth
- 2 heads cauliflower, cored and sliced into florets
- ¼ cup fresh chives, chopped
- ¼ cup Parmesan cheese, grated
- Salt and pepper to taste

Instruction

1. In a pot over medium heat, pour in the chicken broth.
2. Add the cauliflower.
3. Bring to a boil and then simmer for 20 minutes.
4. Transfer cauliflower to a blender. Pulse until smooth.
5. Stir in the chives and cheese.
6. Season with salt and pepper.

Nutrition Per Servings: Kcal: 98, Protein: 9g, Fat: 4g, Net Carb: 6g

Garlic Parmesan Zucchini

Prep. Time: 05 min

Cook Time: 20 min

Servings: 6 People

Ingredients

- ¼ cup Parmesan cheese
- ¼ cup mayonnaise
- 1 clove garlic, minced

- Salt to taste
- 2 zucchinis, sliced

Instruction

1. Preheat your oven to 400 degrees F.
2. Combine all the ingredients except the zucchini.
3. Spread mixture on top of zucchini.
4. Bake in the oven for 20 minutes.

Nutrition Per Servings: Kcal: 80, Protein: 6g, Fat: 4g, Net Carb: 4g

Mashed Cauliflower with Chives

Prep. Time: 15 min

Cook Time: 25 min

Servings: 4 People

Ingredients

- 2 cups chicken broth
- 2 heads cauliflower, cored and sliced into florets
- ¼ cup fresh chives, chopped
- ¼ cup Parmesan cheese, grated
- Salt and pepper to taste

Instruction

1. In a pot over medium heat, pour in the chicken broth.
2. Add the cauliflower.
3. Bring to a boil and then simmer for 20 minutes.
4. Transfer cauliflower to a blender. Pulse until smooth.
5. Stir in the chives and cheese.
6. Season with salt and pepper.

Nutrition Per Servings: Kcal: 98, Protein: 9g, Fat: 4g, Net Carb: 6g

Keto ground beef and green beans

Prep. Time: 10 min

Cook Time: 20 min

Servings: 2 People

Ingredients

- 10 oz. ground beef
- 9 oz. fresh green beans
- 3½ oz. butter
- salt and pepper
- 1/3 cup mayonnaise or crème fraîche (optional)

Instruction

1. Rinse and trim the green beans.
2. Heat up a generous dollop of butter in a frying pan where you can fit both the ground beef and the green beans.
3. Brown the ground beef on high heat until it's almost done. Add salt and pepper.
4. Lower the heat somewhat. Add more butter and fry the beans for 5 minutes in the same pan. Stir the ground beef every now and then.
5. Season beans with salt and pepper. Serve with remaining butter and add mayonnaise or crème fraiche if you need more fat for satiety.

Nutrition Per Servings: Kcal: 698, Protein: 35g, Fat: 60g, Net Carb: 5g

Low-carb baked eggs

Prep. Time: 05 min

Cook Time: 15 min

Servings: 1 People

Ingredients

- 3 oz. ground beef
- 2 eggs
- 2 oz. shredded cheese

Instruction

1. Preheat the oven to 400°F (200°C).

2. Arrange cooked ground-beef mixture in a small baking dish. Then make two holes with a spoon and crack the eggs into them.
3. Sprinkle shredded cheese on top.
4. Bake in the oven until the eggs are done, about 10-15 minutes.
5. Let cool for a while. The eggs and ground meat get very hot!

Nutrition Per Servings: Kcal: 498, Protein: 41g, Fat: 35g, Net Carb: 2g

Butter Hardboiled Eggs

Prep. Time: 05 min

Cook Time: 10 min

Servings: 1 People

Ingredients

- 2 whole Eggs
- 30g Butter
- 1 tbsp Mascarpone
- Salt &pepper to taste

Instruction

1. Hard boil the eggs in a pot. Add a pinch of salt to it so the eggs will peel bet- ter once done.
2. Wash the boiled eggs with cold water. Peel and chop into a large cup.
3. Next, add the mascarpone cheese and butter while the eggs are still hot, mix- ing well. Season with salt and pepper.

Nutrition Per Servings: Kcal: 430, Protein: 14g, Fat: 41g, Net Carb: 1g

Creamy Avocado Cacao Chia Shake

Prep. Time: 01 min

Cook Time: 15 min

Servings: 1 People

Ingredients

- ½ avocado

- 1 tbsp chia seeds
- ½ oz 70% dark chocolate
- 1 cup unsweetened almond milk
- 5 ice cubes

Instruction

1. Mix the chia seeds with the unsweetened almond milk and wait for 10 minutes.
2. Add all the ingredients to the blender.
3. Blend until smooth.
4. Topped with some chopped dark chocolate.

Nutrition Per Servings: Kcal: 533, Protein: 15g, Fat: 37g, Net Carb: 10g

Crispy-Fried Wings

Prep. Time: 5 min

Cook Time: 15 min

Servings: 2 People

Ingredients

- 12 chicken wings, raw &thawed
- 4 tbsp unsalted butter
- 4 tbsp Frank's Red Hot

Instruction

1. Preheat the fryer oil to 275. Dry the wings and fry for 15 minutes
2. Let wings cool to room temperature.
3. Preheat the fryer to 375 and pat wings dry.
4. Fry for another 6 minutes or until skin is taut and golden brown.
5. If desired, mix melted butter and Frank's Red Hot together.
6. Toss the crispy fried wings in the sauce. Serve!

Nutrition Per Servings: Kcal: 686, Protein: 42g, Fat: 55g, Net Carb: 0g

Perfect Family Roast

Prep. Time: 10 min

Cook Time: 50 min

Servings: 8 People

Ingredients

- 1 tsp. Garlic Powder
- 5 lbs. Beef Rib Roast
- 2 tsp. Salt
- 1 tsp. Pepper

Instruction

1. Let the roast attain room temperature for 1 full hour.
2. Next, Preheat oven to 375F then mix together all the spices.
3. Place roast inside a casserole dish or onto a roasting rack and rub with spices.
4. Roast in the oven for 1 hour. Turn oven off completely. Do not open the door but let the roast sit in the oven for 3 hours.
5. 30 to 45 minutes before serving, turn the oven back on to 375F.
6. Take out roast from oven and leave to rest for about 10 minutes then cut and serving.

Nutrition Per Servings: Kcal: 681, Protein: 90g, Fat: 46g, Net Carb: 5g

Peanut Butter Chia Pudding

Prep. Time: 3 h

Cook Time: 00 min

Servings: 1 People

Ingredients

- 1 tbsp chia seeds
- 1 cup unsweetened almond milk
- ½ tsp ground cinnamon
- 1 tbsp peanut butter
- 8 drops stevia

Instruction

1. Add almond milk, peanut butter, cinnamon and stevia to your blender.
2. Blend until smooth.
3. Add chia seeds to the mixture and stir.
4. Refrigerate for about 3 hours.
5. Enjoy!

Nutrition Per Servings: Kcal: 384, Protein: 16.5g, Fat: 25g, Net Carb: 11g

Salted Toffee Walnut Cups

Prep. Time: 20 min

Cook Time: 05 min

Servings: 5 People

Ingredients

- 5 oz milk chocolate, low-carb
- 5 tablespoons erythritol, divided
- 3 tablespoons cold butter
- ½ oz raw walnuts, chopped
- Salt to taste

Instruction

1. Place the chocolate in the microwave and melt at 45- second intervals with frequent stirring.
2. Line a cupcake pan with 5 paper liners and spoon a chocolate into each liner. Spread to cover the bottom evenly and then use a pastry brush or spoon to brush up the chocolate edges a little. Freeze to harden.
3. Combine the erythritol and cold butter in a microwave bowl and heat for 3 minutes, stirring every 30 seconds or so to prevent burning. If mixture is too watery afterwards, thicken with extra 2 teaspoons of erythritol and add the chopped walnuts as well.

4. Take out the chocolate cups from the freezer and if necessary, reheat. Now fill each cup with a spoon of the toffee mixture. Stir slowly and work quickly be- cause the mixture will begin to separate and harden.

5. Top with the rest of the chocolate and refrigerate an hour to cool. 6. Take them out from cups and then sprinkle with salt.

Nutrition Per Servings: Kcal: 194, Protein: 18g, Fat: 2.5g, Net Carb: 2.5g

Keto Milk Chocolate

Prep. Time: 10 min

Cook Time: 20 min

Servings: 13 People

Ingredients

- 5 ounces of cocoa butter
- 5 ounce of baking chocolate, unsweetened, chopped
- 21/2 ounce of powdered erythritol 1ounce of whey protein powder
- 3/4 teaspoon of liquid stevia extract

Instruction

1. Add together the whey protein and erythritol, blending well to combine to fine powder.

2. Melt the cocoa butter, with continuous stirring, in a double boiler or a small pan over low heat.

3. Add the baking chocolate and keep stirring until smooth.

4. Now add the whey protein and erythritol as well as the stevia, while stirring to mix well.

5. Remove from heat and stir to smoothness.

6. Pour into chocolate molds and place in the refrigerator to cool and hard- ened.

7. Enjoy at room temperature.

Nutrition Per Servings: Kcal: 170, Protein: 3g, Fat: 17g, Net Carb: 3.5g

No-Bake Keto Cookies

Prep. Time: 5 min

Cook Time: 5 min

Servings: 18 People

Ingredients

- 2 tablespoons of real butter
- 2/3 cup of peanut butter
- 1 cup of unsweetened coconut, shredded
- 4 drops of vanilla stevia

Instruction

1. Add butter to microwave bowl, place in the microwave and melt.
2. Add peanut butter, stir, and add the sweetener as well as the coconut, mixing well.
3. Transfer to sheet pan and freeze for 5 to 10 minutes.
4. Bag and refrigerate, afterwards.

Nutrition Per Servings: Kcal: 80, Protein: 0g, Fat: 0g, Net Carb: 0g

Caprese Salad

Prep. Time: 10 min

Cook Time: 0 min

Servings: 1 People

Ingredients

- 2 tomatoes, sliced
- ¼ cups fresh basil leaves
- 1 large ball of Mozzarella, sliced
- 3 tbsp olive oil
- Sea salt and black pepper to taste

Instruction

1. In a serving plate, layer the tomatoes, mozzarella and basil.
2. Drizzle with olive oil and sprinkle with salt and black pepper.

3. Enjoy!

Nutrition Per Servings: Kcal: 387, Protein: 1g, Fat: 41g, Net Carb: 3g

Cream Cheese Crepes

Prep. Time: 05 min

Cook Time: 05 min

Servings: 6 People

Ingredients

- 4 egg whites
- 4 eggs
- 4 tablespoons of cream cheese butter
- 2 tablespoons of psyllium husk

Instruction

1. Blend all the ingredients together in a food processor or regular blender.
2. Melt a little butter in a skillet on medium heat.
3. Add some of the batter and then swirl to distribute evenly, pancake style. Cook over until the top is firm then flip and cook on the other side.
4. Repeat until you run out of batter.

Nutrition Per Servings: Kcal: 103, Protein: 7g, Fat: 06g, Net Carb: 3g

Cauliflower Bake

Prep. Time: 10 min

Cook Time: 15 min

Servings: 6 People

Ingredients

- 1 small cauliflower head, grated
- ¾ cup of shredded cheddar cheese
- 1 egg

- ½ teaspoon lemon pepper seasoning
- Salt and black pepper, to taste

Instruction

1. Microwave the grated cauliflower for 3 minutes and leave to cool; add the cooled cauliflower to paper towels and wring until it has no excess water. Put in a bowl.
2. Add the remaining ingredients to the bowl and mix with the cauliflower.
3. Coat a baking pan with nonstick cooking spray.
4. Shape the cauliflower mixture into 6 square or rectangular patties and place on the pan.
5. Bake for 15-20 minutes at 400°F.
6. Remove when done and leave for 10 minutes to cool so it can set.

Nutrition Per Servings: Kcal: 164, Protein: 7g, Fat: 11g, Net Carb: 5g

Zucchini Tomato Soup

Prep. Time: 05 min

Cook Time: 10 min

Servings: 2 People

Ingredients

- 2 large tomatoes, chopped
- 2 fresh basil leaves, for garnish
- 1 medium zucchini, julienned
- 1 teaspoon of olive oil
- 1 garlic clove, crushed

Instruction

1. Add oil to a pan on medium heat.
2. Stir-fry the garlic and zucchini strips for 3-4 minutes.
3. Stir in the tomatoes with its liquid; cook soup for another 3-4 minutes.
4. Ladle soup into bowls and garnish with basil.

Nutrition Per Servings: Kcal: 60, Protein: 2.5g, Fat: 2.5g, Net Carb: 7g

Easy Keto Ice Cream

Prep. Time: 10 min

Cook Time: 30 min

Servings: 1 People

Ingredients

- 4 large eggs
- ¼ tsp cream of tartar
- ½ cup erythritol
- 1¼ cup heavy whipping cream
- 1 tbsp vanilla extract

Instruction

1. Start by separating your egg yolks from your egg whites, and whisk the egg whites with the cream of tartar. The egg whites will begin to thicken, and as they do you're going to need to add the Erythritol. They should start to form stiff peaks, and you'll need to keep whisking until they do.
2. Take another bowl, and start to whisk your cream. Soft peaks should start to form as the whisk is removed, but you'll need to be careful not to over whisk the cream.
3. In a third bowl, combine your egg yolks with the vanilla.
4. Now you can fold the whisked egg whites into the now whipped cream.
5. Add in your egg yolk mixture, and continue to gently fold with a spatula until thoroughly combined.
6. Place it in a pan, preferably a loaf pan, and let it sit. All hands on time is done, but it'll need to sit for about two hours.

Nutrition Per Servings: Kcal: 238, Protein: 5g, Fat: 22g, Net Carb: 2g

Scrambled Eggs with Bacon

Prep. Time: 05 min

Cook Time: 10 min

Servings: 1 People

Ingredients

- 4 slices sugar-free bacon
- 6 large eggs

- ¼ cup heavy cream
- ¼ teaspoon salt
- ¼ teaspoon black pepper

Instruction

1. Cook bacon in a medium skillet over medium heat until crispy, about 10 minutes. Remove bacon from pan and dice.
2. Crack eggs into a medium bowl and whisk together with heavy cream, salt, and pepper. Add egg mixture to bacon grease in pan and stir until scrambled. Add diced bacon to eggs and stir.
3. Remove from heat and serve immediately.

Nutrition Per Servings: Kcal: 324, Protein: 8g, Fat: 35g, Net Carb: 2g

Crispy Chicken Wings

Prep. Time: 10 min

Cook Time: 60 min

Servings: 2 People

Ingredients

- 2 lbs chicken wings
- 1 ½ tbsp baking powder
- 2 tsp salt

Instruction

1. Pat chicken wings dry with a paper towel and place in a plastic bag. Sprinkle with baking powder and salt, and shake to coat.
2. Bake at 250°F or 130°C for 30 minutes.
3. Next, increase oven temperature to 425°F or 220°C and continue to bake for another 20 to 30 minutes, until crispy.
4. Toss in a sauce of your choice and enjoy.

Nutrition Per Servings: Kcal: 592, Protein: 99g, Fat: 16g, Net Carb: 5g

Kale Chips

Prep. Time: 10 min

Cook Time: 05 min

Servings: 2 People

Ingredients

- 3 tsp of olive oil
- 12 pieces of kale leaves
- Salt and pepper, as needed

Instruction

1. Preheat oven to 350°F or 175°C.
2. Line a baking sheet with parchment paper.
3. Wash and thoroughly dry kale leaves and place them on the baking sheet.
4. Drizzle kale with olive oil and sprinkle with salt and pepper.
5. Bake 10 to 15 minutes.
6. Serve.

Nutrition Per Servings: Kcal: 107, Protein: 4g, Fat: 7g, Net Carb: 4g

Keto Pizza Chips

Prep. Time: 10 min

Cook Time: 05 min

Servings: 8 People

Ingredients

- 10 oz sliced pepperoni
- 1 (8 oz) bag shredded mozzarella cheese
- 1 (8 oz) bag shredded Parmesan cheese
- 2 tsp Italian seasoning

Instruction

1. Preheat oven to 400°F or 200°C.
2. Line two cookie sheets with aluminum foil, and place the pepperoni on the sheets.
3. Sprinkle with shredded mozzarella cheese, grated parmesan, and Italian seasoning.
4. Bake for 8-10 minutes.
5. Remove and let cool for about 5 minutes or until crispy.

6. Serve with marinara if you like.

Nutrition Per Servings: Kcal: 250, Protein: 0g, Fat: 18g, Net Carb: 2g

Chia Seeds Smoothie

Prep. Time: 10 min

Cook Time: 00 min

Servings: 2 People

Ingredients

- 4 Tablespoons of Chia seeds
- 2 Cups of Coconut milk (full fat)
- 1/2 Cup of blueberries (frozen)
- 4 Tablespoons of Coconut oil (melted)

Instruction

1. Put the entire ingredients in a blender and blend until combined
2. Serve cold and enjoy

Nutrition Per Servings: 807g, fat: 84.6g, carbs 18.6g, Protein 5.8g, sugar 11.6g

Feta Cheese Omelet

Prep. Time: 05 min

Cook Time: 10 min

Servings: 2 People

Ingredients

- 4 large eggs
- 1/2 teaspoon of black pepper
- 1 teaspoon heavy cream
- 3 tablespoons of crumbled feta cheese
- 1 tablespoon vegetable oil

Instruction

1. Beat eggs with pepper in a small bowl.
2. Combine heavy cream with crumbled cheese in another bowl.

3. Heat oil over medium-high heat in a cast iron skillet. Add beaten eggs and tilt the skillet to cover the bottom evenly.
4. When eggs are set, spoon feta mixture onto the center of the omelet. Use a spatula to fold the eggs on opposite sides to the center, then fold over again.

Nutrition Per Servings: Calories 243, Carbohydrates 2g, Fat 20g, Protein 15g

Sausage and Eggs

Prep. Time: 10 min

Cook Time: 35 min

Servings: 4 People

Ingredients

- 2 cups of chopped sausages
- 1 cup baby spinach
- 1 tablespoon olive oil
- 8 eggs
- 2 tablespoons chopped fresh parsley

Instruction

1. Preheat your oven to 375°F.
2. In a large skillet, heat the oil on medium heat. Add sausages and cook with constant stirring until browned on all sides, about 2 to 3 minutes.
3. Add the spinach and cook for a few minutes more.
4. Whisk the eggs in a bowl then combine with the sausage, spinach and parsley. Season with salt and pepper if desired.
5. Pour everything into a greased 8 by 8-inch pan.
6. Bake at 375°F for 20-25 minutes.

Nutrition Per Servings: Calories 332, Carbohydrates 1.2g, Fat 23g, Protein 27g

Easy Bacon and Eggs

Prep. Time: 05 min

Cook Time: 10 min

Servings: 4 People

Ingredients

- 8 slices bacon
- 8 eggs
- 1 teaspoon garlic powder
- 1 teaspoon onion powder
- Sea salt and pepper to taste

Instruction

1. In a skillet, cook bacon until crisp. Transfer to a plate, leaving the grease in the skillet.
2. Beat the eggs with garlic powder and onion powder then fry in the bacon grease. Season to taste with salt and pepper.

Nutrition Per Servings: Calories 226, Carbohydrates 2g, Fat 17g, Protein 18g

Surprise Recipes

Chicken Curry

Prep. Time: 10 min

Cook Time: 40 min

Servings: 10 People

Ingredients

- 4 chicken breasts cut into bite size
- 1 tablespoon coconut oil
- 8 tablespoons curry powder
- 1 (28-ounce) can crushed tomatoes
- 1 (6-ounce) can unsweetened coconut milk

Instruction

1. Heat coconut oil in a skillet on medium heat. Add chicken pieces and cook until browned.
2. Add the tomatoes and curry powder. Stir to combine and let simmer for 30 minutes.
3. Stir in the coconut milk and let cook for additional 10 minutes.

Nutrition Per Servings: Calories 132, Carbohydrates 5.2g, Fat 3.4g, Protein 16.7g

Easy Baked Chicken Breast

Prep. Time: 05 min

Cook Time: 50 min

Servings: 04 People

Ingredients

- 4 chicken breast quarters
- 1 teaspoon olive oil
- 1 teaspoon of salt

Instruction

1. Loosen the chicken skin then season chicken with salt.
2. Transfer the chicken to an ungreased baking pan then brush generously with oil.
3. Bake, uncovered for 40-50minutes at 325°F.

Nutrition Per Servings: Calories 203, Carbohydrates <1g, Fat 5g, Protein 36g

Garlic Chicken

Prep. Time: 10 min

Cook Time: 10 min

Servings: 04 People

Ingredients

- 3 tablespoons butter
- 4 chicken breast halves, skinless, boneless
- 2 teaspoons garlic powder
- 1 teaspoon onion powder
- 1 teaspoon seasoning salt

Instruction

1. Add the butter to a large skillet and melt on medium high heat.
2. Sprinkle onion powder, garlic powder and seasoning salt all over the chicken.
3. Add chicken to hot butter and cook for 10 to 15 minutes per side, or until cooked through.

Nutrition Per Servings: Calories 214, Carbohydrates 1.7g, Fat 10g, Protein 28g

Rosemary Chicken and Bacon

Prep. Time: 10 min

Cook Time: 20 min

Servings: 04 People

Ingredients

- 4 chicken breast halves, skinless, boneless
- 4 slices of bacon
- 4 teaspoons garlic powder
- Salt and pepper to taste
- 4 sprigs of fresh rosemary

Instruction

1. Preheat your outdoor grill to medium-high heat. Clean the grates and oil them lightly.
2. Place chicken breasts in a bowl and toss with garlic powder, salt and pepper.
3. Place one rosemary sprig on each chicken breast then wrap with a slice of bacon. Hold fast with a toothpick.
4. Transfer to the grill and cook for about 8 minutes per side, or until cooked through.

Nutrition Per Servings: Calories 210, Carbohydrates 2.4g, Fat 8.3g, Protein 30g

Grilled Turkey Burgers

Prep. Time: 10 min

Cook Time: 20 min

Servings: 04 People

Ingredients

- 1 pound ground turkey
- 1 packet dry onion soup mix
- 1/2 cup water
- 1/2 teaspoon salt
- 1/2 teaspoon ground black pepper

Instruction

1. Preheat a grill to high heat. Oil the grates lightly.
2. Add ground turkey and the rest of the ingredients to a large bowl. Use your hands to mix until combined then form into 4 patties.
1. Cook the patties until well done, about 5 to 10 minutes per side.

Nutrition Per Servings: Calories 196, Carbohydrates 6.7g, Fat 9g, Protein 23.7g

Spicy Chicken Wings

Prep. Time: 15 min

Cook Time: 45 min

Servings: 04 People

Ingredients

- 20 chicken wings, separated at joints, tips removed
- 1/2 cup red pepper sauce
- 1/2 cup butter, melted
- 1 1/2 tablespoons chili powder
- 3/4 cup tomato sauce

Instruction

1. Preheat your oven to 375°F.
2. Combine the red pepper sauce, butter, chili powder and tomato sauce in a large bowl. Add the wings to the sauce and toss to coat.
3. Bake in the oven until cooked through, about 45 minutes.

Nutrition Per Servings: Calories 411, Carbohydrates 5.1g, Fat 36g, Protein 21g

Juicy Beef Tenderloin

Prep. Time: 05 min

Cook Time: 45 min

Servings: 06 People

Ingredients

- 3 pounds beef tenderloin roast
- 1/2 cup butter, melted
- 3/4 cup soy sauce

Instruction

1. Preheat the oven to 350°F.
2. Place the meet into a shallow, glass baking dish. Pour melted butter and soy sauce over the roast.
3. Bake in the oven for 20 minutes, turn over then continue cooking for another 20 to 25 minutes, occasionally basting with the juices.
4. Remove from oven and let sit for 15 minutes then slice.

Nutrition Per Servings: Calories 593, Carbohydrates 2.5g, Fat 34g, Protein 63.8g

Easy Pork Steaks

Prep. Time: 05 min

Cook Time: 40 min

Servings: 06 People

Ingredients

- 1/4 cup of butter
- 1/4 cup of soy sauce
- 2 garlic cloves, minced
- 1 bunch of green onions
- 6 pork butt steaks

Instruction

1. Melt butter in a large skillet then stir in soy sauce. Add garlic and green onions and cook until lightly browned.
2. Add pork steaks to the skillet. Cover the pan and cook for about 8 to 10 minutes. Turn pork steaks and cook on the other side for another 8 to 10 minutes.
3. Remove the cover and cook for 10 more minutes or until pork steaks are cooked through.

Nutrition Per Servings: Calories 353, Carbohydrates 4g, Fat 25g, Protein 27g

Pure Indulgence Peanut Butter Biscuits

Prep Time: 5 min
Cook Time: 15 min
Servings: 6 People

Ingredients:

- 1 cup almond flour.
- ½ cup peanut butter (unsweetened).
- ⅓ cup erythritol.
- 1 tbsp coconut oil.
- ¾ tsp baking powder.
- ½ tsp vanilla extract.

Instructions:

1. Preheat oven at 350 degrees.
2. In a large bowl, mix all of the ingredients until a dough is formed.
3. Divide the dough into eight large biscuits.
4. Line a baking tray with greaseproof paper.
5. Bake for 10-12 minutes or until golden brown.

Nutrition Per Serving: Fat:16g, Carbohydrates: 6g, Protein: 7g, Calories: 189,

Craftily Creamy Chocolate Mousse

Prep Time: 5 min
Cook Time: 15 min
Servings: 2 People

Ingredients:

- 3 oz cream cheese.
- ½ cup of thick cream.
- ¼ cup powdered sweetener.
- 2 tbsp cocoa powder.
- 1 tsp vanilla extract.
- Pinch of salt.

Instructions:

1. In a blender, mix the cream cheese until soft and fluffy.
2. Slowly add in the thick cream, vanilla extract, sweetener, cocoa powder, and salt.
3. Mix until well blended and soft and fluffy.
4. Chill in the fridge for 30 minutes.

Nutrition Per Serving: Fat: 38g, Carbohydrates: 6.5g, Protein: 7g, Calories: 372

Chewy Coconut Chunks

Prep Time: 10 min
Cook Time: 35 min
Servings: 8 People

Ingredients:

- 7 oz coconut (shredded).
- ⅔ cup coconut milk (full fat).
- ¼ cup maple syrup.
- 1 tsp psyllium husk.
- ¼ tsp almond extract.
- ¼ tsp salt.

Instructions:

1. Preheat oven at 325 degrees.
2. In a blender, mix coconut milk, maple syrup, psyllium husk, almond extract, salt, and ¾ of the coconut flakes until smooth.
3. Pour mixture into a large bowl, stir in remaining coconut flakes.
4. Line a baking tray with greaseproof paper. Using a tablespoon, scoop out chunks of the mixture and place onto the plate.
5. Bake for 30 minutes or until all chunks are golden brown.

Nutrition Per Serving: Fat: 10g, Carbohydrates: 7g, Protein: 2g, Calories: 111

Keto chicken enchilada bowl

Prep Time: 10 min
Cook Time: 25 min
Servings: 4 People

Ingredients:

- Two tablespoon coconut oil (for searing chicken)
- 1 pound of boneless, skinless chicken thighs
- 3/4 cup red enchilada sauce (recipe from Low Carb Maven)
- 1/4 cup water
- 1/4 cup chopped onion
- 1– 4 oz can dice green chiles

Instructions:

1. In a pot or dutch oven over medium heat, melt the coconut oil. Once hot, sear chicken thighs until lightly brown.
2. Pour in enchilada sauce and water, then add onion and green chiles. Reduce heat to a simmer and cover. Cook chicken for 17-25 minutes or until chicken is tender and fully cooked through to at least 165 degrees internal temperature.
3. Carefully removes the chicken and place it onto a work surface. Chop or shred chicken (your preference), then add it back into the pot. Let the chicken simmer uncovered for an additional 10 minutes to absorb flavour and allow the sauce to reduce a little.
4. To serve, top with avocado, cheese, jalapeno, sour cream, tomato, and any other desired toppings. Feel free to customize these to your preference. Serve alone or over cauliflower rice, if desired, just be sure to update your nutrition info as needed.

Nutrition Per Serving: Calories: 568, Calories Fat: 40.21g, Protein: 38.38g, Fat: 40.21g

Healthy Lunchtime Ham & Cheese Wrap

Prep Time: 10 min
Cook Time: 15 min
Servings: 2 People

Ingredients:

- 5 iceberg lettuce leaves.
- Four slices sandwich ham.
- 4 slices cheddar cheese.
- ¼ cup guacamole.
- One tomato (sliced).
- ½ red onion (finely sliced.

Instructions:

1. Layer lettuce leaves onto a sheet of cling film. Ensure the leaves overlap with each other.
2. Layer the ham and cheese onto the leaves.
3. Do the same with tomato and onion and finally top with guacamole.
4. Using the clingfilm (as if you were using a sushi mat), roll the lettuce tightly to make the wrap.
5. When completely rolled, cut the wrap in half.

Nutrition Per Serving: Fat: 31g, Carbohydrates: 14g, Protein: 33g, Calories: 459

Cheesy Chicken Chunks

Prep Time: 10 min
Cook Time: 10 min
Servings: 3 People

Ingredients:

- 2 large chicken breasts (cut into strips).
- One large egg.
- ¾ cup parmesan cheese (grated).
- ¾ cup almond flour.

Instructions:

1. Preheat oven at 400 degrees.
2. Mix the parmesan and flour.
3. In a separate bowl, whisk the egg.
4. Dip each strip of chicken into the egg mixture and then into the flour mixture. Place on a wire rack.
5. Spray chicken with cooking spray and bake for 18-20 minutes or until browned and thoroughly cooked.

Nutrition Per Serving: Fat: 24g, Carbohydrates: 2g, Protein: 41g, Calories: 398

Creamy Avocado Cilantro

Prep Time: 10 min
Cook Time: 5 min
Servings: 5 People

Ingredients:

- One avocado split and pitted
- ½ cup low-fat Greek yoghurt
- One clove garlic minced
- juice of 1 lime
- 2 tbsp cilantro chopped
- salt and Pepper to taste

Instructions:

1. In a small bowl, whisk together lime juice, olive oil, garlic, chilli powder, cumin, paprika, salt, pepper, red pepper flakes. Pour into a resealable bag and add shrimp. Toss to coat and marinate for 30 minutes.
2. Preheat the grill to medium heat. Put the shrimp on skewers and place on the rack—grill on each side for about two minutes or until no longer pink.
3. To make the creamy avocado cilantro sauce add the avocado, greek yoghurt, garlic, lime, and cilantro. Pulse in a food processor until smooth. Add salt and Pepper to taste. Serve immediately with shrimp.

Nutrition Per Serving: Cholesterol 1mg, Sodium 215mg, Potassium 13mg, Fiber 1g, Sugar 1g

Spain Cheesy-Meat Tapas

Prep Time: 10 min
Cook Time: 10 min
Servings: 2 People

Ingredients:

- 8 oz prosciutto (sliced).
- 8 oz chorizo (sliced).
- 4 oz cheddar cheese (cubed).
- 4 oz mozzarella (cubed).
- 4 oz cucumber (cubed).
- 2 oz red pepper (sliced).

Instructions:

1. Arrange all items on a plate.
2. Enjoy.

Nutrition Per Serving: Fat: 74g, Carbohydrates: 8g, Protein: 57g, Calories: 944

Tasty Salted Turnip Fries

Prep Time: 10 min
Cook Time: 10 min
Servings: 2 People

Ingredients:

- 16 oz turnips.
- 6 tbsp olive oil.
- 2 tsp onion powder.
- ½ tsp paprika.
- 1 tsp salt.

Instructions:

1. Preheat oven at 400 degrees.
2. Wash and peel the turnips; cut into ½ inch strips.
3. In a large bowl, toss the turnips in 2 tbsp of olive oil, salt, onion powder, and paprika.
4. Add remaining oil to a baking tray and heat in the oven for 5 minutes.
5. Bake for 25-30 minutes or until fries are golden brown and crispy.

Nutrition Per Serving: Fat: 22g, Carbohydrates: 7g, Protein: 2g, Calories: 219

Overnight Oats

Prep Time: 5 min
Cook Time: 10 min
Servings: 3 People

Ingredients:

- 1 cup organic rolled oats
- 2 ½ cups Strawberry Cashew Milk
- 1 Tablespoon Chia seeds
- 1 Tablespoon Whole flax seeds

Instructions:

1. Place rolled oats, chia seeds, and flax seeds in a large bowl. Poor in 2 ½ cups of strawberry cashew milk (or preferred dairy, nut or seed milk) and stir well to combine. Cover and store in the fridge for 1 hour or overnight.
2. Check consistency and add additional Strawberry Cashew Milk as desired. Portion into individual containers. Add fresh strawberries, cashews, chia seeds, flax seeds, or extra Strawberry Cashew Milk as toppings. Enjoy immediately or store in airtight containers for up to 5 days.

Nutrition Per Serving: Fat: 70g, Carbohydrates: 35g, Protein: 15g, Calories: 533,

CONCLUSION

I will definitely keep the final thought of this resource short, yet there are a few factors I wish to stress anyway.

The keto diet plan concentrates greatly on reducing carbohydrates and maximizing fatty acids, but only the nutritious ones. I am confident that, by now, you have knowledge of the huge difference between really good fats and things like trans fats.

This kind of diet might just be the most crucial choice you've ever made. Many thanks for everything! I appreciate you making the effort to read my book. It took me a very long time to put it together, so can I just ask you to write a brief customer review? This way, others will learn what you thought about it.

Dr. Daniel Smith

Thank you for buying this book. If you have 30 seconds, please share your thoughts and leave a review. Thanks again.

Printed in Great Britain
by Amazon